Understanding Patient Safety: Volume 2

Understanding Patient Safety: Volume 2

Susy Cowen

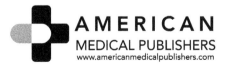

AMERICAN
MEDICAL PUBLISHERS
www.americanmedicalpublishers.com

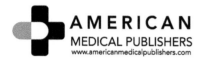
AMERICAN
MEDICAL PUBLISHERS
www.americanmedicalpublishers.com

Cataloging-in-publication Data

Understanding patient safety : volume 2 / Susy Cowen.
    p. cm.
Includes bibliographical references and index.
ISBN 979-8-88740-545-2
1. Patients--Safety measures. 2. Patients--Care. 3. Medical errors--Prevention.
4. Medicine--Practice--Safety measures. I. Cowen, Susy.
R729.8 .U53 2023
610.289--dc23

American Medical Publishers,
41 Flatbush Avenue,
1st Floor, New York,
NY 11217, USA

ISBN 979-8-88740-545-2 (Hardback)

Contents

Preface

Patient safety refers to a health care discipline that evolved in response to the increasing complexity of health care systems and the consequent increase of patient harm in health care facilities. The goal of patient safety is to prevent and minimize harm, risks and errors while providing health care services to patients. It majorly focuses on the continuous improvement which is based on learning from adverse events and errors. Patient safety is critical to provide high-quality health services. Skilled health care personnel, clear policies, patient involvement, data to drive safety improvements and leadership ability are all required for supporting successful implementation of patient safety methods. There are various situations which are concerned with patient safety, such as unsafe injections practices, radiation errors, venous thromboembolism, medication errors, diagnostic errors, health care-associated infections, unsafe transfusion practices and unsafe surgical care procedures. This book provides significant information to help develop a good understanding of patient safety. Its extensive content provides the readers with a thorough understanding of the subject.

The researches compiled throughout the book are authentic and of high quality, combining several disciplines and from very diverse regions from around the world. Drawing on the contributions of many researchers from diverse countries, the book's objective is to provide the readers with the latest achievements in the area of research. This book will surely be a source of knowledge to all interested and researching the field.

In the end, I would like to express my deep sense of gratitude to all the authors for meeting the set deadlines in completing and submitting their research chapters. I would also like to thank the publisher for the support offered to us throughout the course of the book. Finally, I extend my sincere thanks to my family for being a constant source of inspiration and encouragement.

Susy Cowen

Part III
Major Challenges and their Solutions

18

Doctors and their Challenging Duty Hours

On March 5, 1984, Bennington College freshman Libby Zion died at New York Hospital. She had been admitted the night before with vague symptoms and strange jerking motions. After consulting with her family physician, the residents on call gave her intravenous solutions for possible dehydration and prescribed meperidine to control her jerking motions. They then left to take care of other patients. Luise Weinstein, the first-year resident, was responsible for 40 other patients. No sleep for her.

Libby Zion did not improve; she became more agitated. Weinstein ordered restraints, which Zion fought against. Finally, she went to sleep. But her temperature rose, and by 6:30 AM it reached 107 °F. Weinstein took measures to cool her down, but she quickly deteriorated, had a cardiac arrest, and could not be resuscitated.

Her father, Sidney Zion, a lawyer and a writer for the New York Times, was furious. He was convinced her death was due to inadequate care by poorly supervised, overworked residents. In a *New York Times* op-ed piece, he wrote: "You don't need kindergarten to know that a resident working a 36-hour shift is in no condition to make any kind of judgment call—forget about life-and-death." He decried the lack of supervision of the residents and accused the doctors of murder. He launched an unremitting public campaign for justice [1].

A full investigation later concluded that the probable cause of death was a reaction between the prescribed meperidine and an antidepressant she was taking, phenelzine. This interaction was not well-known, and, in fact, at a hearing 2 years later several chairmen of departments of medicine at prominent medical schools stated they had never heard of the interaction prior to this case.

Sidney Zion pursued the legal challenge, however, and in 1986 a grand jury charged the residents with negligence. However, after multiple reviews and conflicting findings by state regulatory bodies over several years, an appeals court in 1991 cleared them of all charges [2]. Zion then filed a civil suit which in 1995 concluded with a judgment that the primary care physician and the residents pay Zion $375,000 [2].

Residency Training

The system for training doctors goes back to the 1890s, when William Stewart Halsted, the professor of surgery at the Johns Hopkins Hospital, formalized the training of surgeons. Halsted believed that total immersion in the care of patients was the best way to learn about disease and treatment and to develop a sense of commitment to the patient.

After completing medical school, surgical trainees at Hopkins were required to literally live at the hospital—the origin of the term "resident"—and were discouraged from marrying. Supervised by senior physicians called "Attending Physicians," they were responsible for all aspects of care, including menial tasks such as drawing blood for tests, changing dressings, and transporting patients for tests. It was a long process: up to 10 years for some.

Other specialties adopted the residency concept, gradually modifying it to require 30 hours in-hospital on alternate days, the custom at the time of the Libby Zion case. Surgical training typically required 5 years, medical specialties, three. Residents (also called "house officers") were not paid for their services—after all, they were getting a free education—but they got free uniforms and room and board while in the hospital.

Although they were budding professionals, hospitals often treated them like military academy plebes. An apocryphal story that I heard while a surgical resident at the Massachusetts General Hospital many years later was that a former hospital director was so incensed with residents standing around with their hands in their pockets that he had the pockets of their uniforms sewn shut!

The number of residencies increased as the number of specialties expanded dramatically in the mid-twentieth century. In addition to supervised clinical experience and bedside teaching, programs provided teaching conferences. Few residents were paid anything until the 1960s, when they began to receive a meager "stipend" to meet personal expenses—nothing for living expenses outside the hospital, such as food and rent. Hospitals found it convenient to ignore the reality that now most residents were married, and some had children.

Forty years later, in 2001, the mean salary for residents was $40,000 a year, an average of $9.61 an hour for the typical 80-hour week [3]. Residents' expertise, skills, and dedication enable faculty at teaching hospitals to take care of very sick and complicated patients without hiring help or needing to be present all the time. The "purpose" of residency training may be education, but its practical effect—and attraction for the hospital and its doctors—is the 24/7 service doctors in training provide at below minimum wages.

The sleep deprivation and high workloads of busy acute clinical care practice pose a threat to patient safety for any physician, but especially for residents during training. It has been demonstrated, and we all know from personal experience, that judgment and performance suffer when we are up all night or are excessively fatigued from overwork. There is no reason to believe that physicians have some special immunity to these effects. Other critical industries such as commercial aviation and nuclear power recognize the effects of sleep deprivation and strictly limit work hours. Why should medicine be different? The Zion case forced the public and the profession to confront these issues.

Early History—What Happened After Zion

Following the grand jury indictment in 1986, Health Commissioner David Axelrod (the same person who later funded the Harvard Medical Practice Study) established a blue-ribbon committee headed by Bertrand Bell, the "Bell Commission," to investigate the training and supervision of doctors. It recommended limiting resident work hours and improving supervision [4].

In 1989 New York State adopted the Commission's recommendations and legislated that residents could not work more than 80 hours a week or more than 24 consecutive hours. It also required that they have round-the-clock supervision by attending physicians. Two hundred million dollars was appropriated to hire additional ancillary help and board-certified physicians to assist New York hospitals in compliance [5, 6].

It is worth noting that although it is broadly accepted, the 80-hour limit was not at the time evidence-based. Later studies showed, however, that working more than 80 hours was linked to increased depression, suicide, and needlestick injuries of residents.

On the national level, the professional organization responsible for oversight of most residency and fellowship training programs, the Accreditation Council for Graduate Medical Education (ACGME), took notice. The ACGME is a private, not-for-profit organization that sets standards for US graduate medical training (residency and fellowship) programs and accredits training programs based on compliance with these standards. A resident must successfully complete training in an accredited institution to be eligible for certification in their specialty and licensure to practice.

Within ACGME, resident duty hour standards are set across all specialties by the Board of Directors in concert with the chairs of the 30 specialty review committees in the *common program requirements*. Additional specific and more detailed standards are proposed by the individual Residency Review Committees for each specialty. In addition, there are many subspecialties (such as gastroenterology, nephrology, and cardiology in Internal Medicine) that propose their own standards. In 2018, there were approximately 830 ACGME-accredited institutions sponsoring approximately 11,200 residency and fellowship programs in 180 specialties and subspecialties [7].

In 1988, ACGME spoke up with whispered voice to suggest limiting call to every third night and to permit—not require—its individual specialty Residency Review Committees to incorporate requirements related to work hours in their standards. It did not mandate, as part of the shared requirements, that all specialties adopt a common standard. Not surprisingly, its general request had limited effect. Over the next 2 years, only six specialties—none of them surgical—instituted a limit of 80 hours per week.

New York State did little better. With over 100 teaching hospitals, its hospitals train 15% of the resident physicians in the USA, but it did not initially vigorously enforce its 1989 regulations. This led New York City Public Advocate, Mark Green, in 1994 and 1997 to investigate compliance and report widespread violations. A Department of Health survey in 1998 of 12 hospitals in New York City found that 37% of residents worked more than allowed and 77% of surgical residents worked more than 95 hours per week [8]. The state fined four hospitals $20,000 each and increased the maximum fine to $50,000. Two years later, the state funded and issued a contract for monitoring hospitals and fining them for noncompliance [9].

The pressure for reform continued to build. In April 2001, the NYC residents' union, the Committee of Interns and Residents of the SEIU (CIR), the Public Citizen Health Research Group, the American Medical Student Association, and Dr. Bertrand Bell, petitioned the Occupational Safety and Health Administration to establish and enforce a federal work hour standard for residents [10]. It didn't happen.

In November 2001, a bill was introduced in the House of Representatives to limit work hours of residents to 80 hours a week and to provide for federal enforcement [11]. Meanwhile, the Association of American Medical Colleges (AAMC) issued a policy statement recommending limits on work hours. The ACGME became more active in enforcement; in 2002 it withdrew accreditation of the general surgery program at Yale-New Haven Medical Center because of excessive work hours [12]. Finally, seeking to forestall the pending federal regulation, the ACGME decided it was time to act.

2003 ACGME Regulations

In 2002 the ACGME announced new regulations of resident hours and workloads, to take effect July 1, 2003 [13]. Although most people had seen it coming, it still aroused great consternation. The ACGME had already gradually stiffened requirements, limiting overnight on-call duty to every third night and requiring residents to have 1 day off every 7 days worked. A number of non-surgical specialties had imposed an 80-hour work week limit.

The surgeons, however, had rejected the hour limits. The Residency Review Committee for Surgery gave hospital surgical program directors responsibility for "appropriate" duty hours. They stressed that continuity of care must take precedence without regard to time of day, call schedules, or number of hours already worked. Work weeks of 100–120 hours were still common [14, 15].

The new regulations made the 80-hour week mandatory for all specialties and added a 24-hour limit for on-call duty. Hospitals were required to monitor work hours and reduce residents' responsibility for patient care support services of no educational value, such as drawing blood for tests, starting intravenous lines, and transporting patients [16]. The ACGME would monitor compliance.

These stronger standards, however, fell short of the AMA and AAMC recommendations for shorter on-call hours, or those in the legislation proposed by Congress. Nonetheless, both the AMA and the AAMC endorsed the changes. The new rules were met with skepticism from CIR, Public Citizen, and the New York Times [17]. They also aroused strong feels within the profession—pro and con—the latter especially among the surgeons.

The Duty Hours Debate

The arguments for hour and workload limitations are basically two: that it will reduce injuries and that it will improve residents' mental health and well-being. The evidence of the potential harm to patients from sleep deprivation is abundant. Many studies over the years of its effects on various populations have shown the risk of sleep deprivation [18, 19], including a memorable study that demonstrated that impairment of performance after 24 hours of sustained wakefulness is equivalent to having a blood alcohol concentration of 0.10% [20].

Specific studies of medical residents' performance also confirm its ill effects [21]. One controlled study of first year residents showed that those with 24-hour sleep deprivation made 36% more serious errors than those who worked 16 hour days, and they made over 5 times as many serious diagnostic errors [22]. Other studies showed residents made twice as many mistakes detecting cardiac arrhythmias when sleep deprived and twice as many technical errors in simulated laparoscopic surgery [23].

A survey of residents showed that 41% reported fatigue as a cause of serious mistakes; of those, 31% were fatal [22]. A meta-analysis of

studies by the ACGME found that after 24–30 hours of sleep deprivation, clinical performance of residents dropped from the 50th to the
7th percentile of performance when rested [24].

Sleep deprivation is also hazardous to the residents themselves.
During night call, they are twice as likely to suffer a needlestick injury
[25]. Driving home after an "all-nighter," the chance they will sustain
a motor vehicle crash that injures the resident or others is increased by
168% [26], and the risk that the accident will be fatal is also increased.

The second argument in favor of shorter hours is that resident well-
being is enhanced. Learning is improved by the fact that residents are
sufficiently awake and alert to benefit both from clinical experience
and from formal educational activities. It was a common experience
for residents to fall asleep during conferences or sometimes even
while standing on rounds. (Your author remembers having this
experience.)

Mood is also improved. Fatigue increases depression, anxiety, confusion, and anger that lead to detachment and lack of compassion for
patients [21]. With adequate rest, attitudes and overall mental health
improve. Finally, more humane hours permit the resident to maintain
a balance between personal and professional lives, which would give
them a better attitude toward their work and their patients.

The arguments against the proposed limits came largely from the
general surgeons and surgical specialists, who raised issues of learning and responsibility. They were concerned that disruption of continuity of care by shorter work hours and more frequent shifts would
deprive the trainee of the opportunity to see a clinical episode evolve
and participate in all aspects of care [27]. Residents would miss
important learning opportunities. They would not participate in
enough operations to develop the needed skills and judgment.

They held out the specter of a surgical resident being forced to drop
out of an operation because his time was up. They decried "shift medicine." They worried that young surgeons wouldn't develop a sense of
responsibility for their patients. Following the patient through the
night and when fatigued was, they maintained, essential to the incul-
cation of accountability and professionalism [27]. Others agreed:
these are critical issues; their fears were justified.

Surgical residents also agreed. They live for the operating room. As
we used to joke when I was a surgical resident, "The only problem

with being on every other night is that you miss half of the good cases." It is difficult for the public or non-surgical physicians to fully appreciate the nature of surgical residency or its allure for residents. Participating in a surgical operation is an exhilarating experience. You see inside the human body, handle its organs, and restore its integrity by removing disease or repairing an injury. There is nothing like it in the world.

Surgical residents want to be able to do it themselves, and they can see they need to practice—a lot. They become almost obsessive about "doing more cases." Like all doctors, they want to do a good job, to become competent. They are willing to pay the price in high work-loads and long hours, although they worry about its effect on their ability to give good care. A surgical resident once shared her feelings with me, "The thing wrong with having too many patients is that it keeps me from giving them the best care possible."

Years later, surgeons still have strong feelings about their residency years. They look back with nostalgia at the long hours, midnight operations, and heroic efforts to save the life of a badly injured trauma victim. They learned by doing, and it was exciting. In retrospect, some may resent the time it took away from their families, but they have no question it was worth it. These experiences reinforce their mindset about training. As we see daily on the political scene, once established, mindsets are hard to change. Evidence, facts, and even compelling contradictory data don't do it.

Other concerns were that the residents would not have time for reading and reflecting on what they were learning from their clinical experience and that shorter shifts would require more frequent hand-offs of care to another doctor, which would cause *more* errors [27]. These were all important issues that needed to be addressed.

Interestingly, in the debate that followed, no one brought up the fact that most countries in the European Union follow its recommendations of a maximum of 48 hours per week and 13 hours maximum shifts. Are European surgeons poorly trained? Do they have poorer outcomes? There is no evidence they do.

But implementing the new rules would require substantial adjustments by hospitals. The purpose of residency training may be education, but residents also provide many services for the hospital that are of no educational value that can be performed by those with far less training. Eliminating these non-educational services was now essential—and long overdue. Filling the gap by hiring more residents was not an option since CMS would not likely fund it. The choices were to increase the workloads of the attendings or to hire more doctors and physician's assistants. A 1994 study estimated that the national cost of these changes would be $1.4–1.8 billion [28].

Some, however, saw that redesigning the system of care to shift resident responsibilities to others would provide an opportunity to better align clinical responsibilities with other educational needs and to rethink the nature of the workplace. The burgeoning patient safety movement was making clear that health-care organizations badly needed to reform their work practices and change their attitudes toward work. It was time to recognize exhaustion not as a sign of dedication but as a risk to patient safety [21].

Regarding responsibility and dedication, Jeff Drazen, editor of the NEJM pointed out, "The role models that trainees see and the integrity of the environment in which they work appear to be far more important for instilling the professional ethos than the duration of the on-call schedules." [27]

What Happened: 2003–2008

Sadly, few surgical training programs and hospitals saw it that way. Most did not see the requirements as an opportunity to improve graduate medical education, but as a threat to the status quo. They refused to change. However, the ACGME required programs to report compliance based on regular reports by the residents of the hours they worked.

The residents were in a bind two ways. If they reported longer hours than permitted, they would incur the ire of their supervisors, jeopardizing both their clinical experience and recommendations for positions after training. And if the program was found in violation, it could lose its accreditation, making the resident ineligible to become board-certified. Program directors made it clear that they expected the reports to show compliance. So residents falsified their reports.

The extent of this deception came to light in 2006, when the Harvard Work Hours Study Group published the results of a confidential study of reporting by first year residents in 700 programs. It showed gross discrepancies: 83.6% reported work hours that were in violation of the ACGME standards. Working shifts greater than 30 consecutive hours was reported by 67.4%, working more than 80 hours a week was reported by 43%, and 43.7% reported not having 1 day in 7 off duty [29].

The ACGME, however, relying on the "official" reports from the program directors reported near-universal compliance with the ACGME standards during the same reporting period, maintaining that only 5.0% of programs were not compliant and that only 3.3% of residents reported violations of the 80-hour rule [29].

Apparently, the leaders of some Residency Review Committees were concerned about responsibility, continuity, and dedication, but it was okay for program directors to force residents to lie. The new rules weren't being observed, and everyone knew it.

The IOM Panel

Other forces were at work. As noted, a series of research studies had emerged that documented the effects of sleep deprivation on errors and harm to patients [26] and harm to residents [25, 26]. Other studies showed that shorter work hours reduced serious medical errors [22, 30, 31] and improved residents' health and education [32]. The CIR continued to press for enforcement. Congress again took notice. In 2007, the House Committee on Energy and Commerce, responding to the evidence linking medical errors to sleep deprivation and overwork and noncompliance with hour limits, requested the IOM to conduct a study and make recommendations.

The IOM convened a distinguished panel of patient safety and quality experts, policy makers, consumer representatives, physicians, nurses, and program directors, who deliberated and had hearings over an 18-month period. In December 2008 it issued its report, *Resident duty hours: Enhancing sleep, supervision and safety* [33]. The IOM called for new measures that would (1) focus not just on the number of hours worked, but on alleviating fatigue and loss of sleep, (2) increase supervision by senior physicians, (3) improve processes for transferring responsibilities from physicians going off duty to those coming on, and (4) stiffen enforcement by initiating federal oversight of the ACGME regulations [33].

It also called on programs not to reduce hours without putting sufficient funding and resources in place to allow for the reduction of hours without overburdening those residents left behind in the hospital. It estimated the total additional cost at $1.7 billion per year.

The IOM Committee took special aim at violations of current duty hour rules, noting that non-adherence to duty hours "is substantial and underreported, and that more intensified monitoring is necessary immediately." It noted "residents fail to accurately report their duty hours for multiple reasons, including fear of repercussions from their supervisors or, at the extreme, fear of causing a training program to lose its accreditation."

It called on the ACGME to address this issue by making unannounced audits of duty hour compliance and implementing protection for whistleblowers. It called on CMS to conduct periodic reviews of ACGME's duty hour monitoring and on the Joint Commission to include adherence data in its surveys and accreditation process.

The IOM's specific recommendations were built on the existing regulations and were consistent with the lessons learned from sleep research and recent studies of residents' work. It called for a maximum of 80 hours duty a week, no more than 16 hours without sleep, maximum on-call duty one night in 3, one full day off each week and 48 hours off once a month, 12 hours off after a night shift, and 48 hours off after 3 or 4 consecutive nights.

The IOM had spoken. The report was hailed not just for the duty hours standards but also for its emphasis on supervision of residents and external oversight of the ACGME. In addition to the IOM panel recommendations, there was mounting public pressure to do something. People were concerned about being harmed by a sleep-deprived doctor. How would the ACGME respond?

ACGME Duty Hour Task Force

We would soon see. When the ACGME implemented its first set of regulations in 2003, it promised a 5-year review. That time had come, and, with the IOM report and the continuing threat of Federal regulation, the ACGME needed to act. In 2008, it commissioned a 16-member Duty Hours Task Force composed of its members, trustees, medical educators, and a consumer, to review relevant research, hear testimony, and draft new standards.

There was concern that limited hours had created a "shift mentality" that conflicted with the physician's moral and professional responsibility to the patient, that programs' focus on duty hours diverted their attention from making needed changes in the learning environment, and that residents were conflicted about leaving patients to comply with the rules [34].

The Task Force discussed the need for enhanced supervision and faculty oversight, improving handovers, and the need to increase attention to patient safety. Research showed that the 2003 regulations had not led to increased hours of sleep. It also showed that reduced hours had no effect on mortality.

Regarding hours, would they heed the IOM recommendations? The leadership was ready to move. The Council of Review Committee Chairs was not so sure. The early signs were not encouraging. At the ACGME June 2009 Congress devoted to duty hours, many representatives of specialty societies spoke out against implementing the IOM recommendations.

Harvard Conference on Duty Hours

Meanwhile, many safety leaders thought the IOM recommendations deserved a broader review, with input not just from leaders of graduate medical education but also from those most affected: patients and residents, nurses, hospitals, and training directors, as well as policy makers and others. The changes proposed by the IOM would affect hundreds of thousands of physicians and residents, over 1000 hospitals, and have a global budget in the billions [35]. Implementing them would be a huge challenge.

The organized voice of residents, the CIR/SEIU, representing 13,000 residents in New York, was particularly concerned about what the ACGME would do. To put pressure on hospitals to implement the IOM recommendations regardless of what the ACGME required, they thought a persuasive strategy would be to provide advice from experts and evidence from those who had successfully implemented hours and workload changes.

At CIR's behest and funding, the leaders of sleep science and resident hours research, Chuck Czeisler and Chris Landrigan, and I convened a 2-day work hours conference at Harvard Medical School in June 2010, *"Enhancing sleep, supervision and safety: What will it take to implement the Institute of Medicine recommendations?"*

Attendees included quality improvement experts, medical educators, hospital administrators, consumers, regulators, sleep scientists, patient advocates, policy makers, a resident, a medical student, and two members of the IOM committee that produced the report. We also had representatives from AHRQ, JCAHO, CMS, and AHA, as well as training directors who had successfully implemented changes in their training programs to meet the 2003 requirements.

A recent survey had shown the disconnect between public perception and reality. The vast majority of the public had no idea that doctors worked 24 hours or more without sleep. When informed of this, only 1% supported it. Eighty percent supported a limit of 16 hours. Importantly, 81% believed that the patient should be informed if the doctor treating them had been working for more than 24 hours: 80% would want a different doctor. Ninety one percent favored strict rules to assure direct on-site supervision by attendings [36].

Roundtable discussions were held on eight topics: workload and supervision, work hours, moonlighting, physician safety, handovers and quality improvement, monitoring and oversight of the ACGME, financial support for implementation, and future research. The head of ACGME, Tom Nasca, himself a supporter of more humane working conditions, addressed the group.

The most memorable feature of the conference was the presentation of three case studies by training directors of programs in internal medicine, obstetrics, and surgery who had successfully developed new programs that functioned well within the hour limits. They showed that the objectives of training could be met and that residents attended more conferences and had higher morale. Both residents and faculty at these institutions were pleased with the results.

In its report, *Implementing the 2009 Institute of Medicine Recommendations on Resident Physician Work Hours, Supervision, and Safety*, the conference made 27 recommendations of necessary and practical steps that are needed to make the new limits work [35]. It concluded that innovators had demonstrated that hours and workloads can be reduced without compromising clinical experience or inhibiting the learning of responsibility, but regulation and financial incentives were needed to facilitate spread.

The ACGME Response

Just a week after the conference, on June 23, 2010, the ACGME Duty Hours Task Force issued its recommendations. It rejected most of the IOM duty hour recommendations except for a maximum duty period of 16 hours for first-year residents (only) and on-site supervision of first-year residents by faculty [34].

The 80-hour work week was retained, as well as limiting on-call duty to every third day (except for "night floats," who were limited to six consecutive nights), and 24 hours off duty every 7 days. However, there was a loophole: programs could apply to be more "flexible" in integrating service with teaching, which could include increasing work hours to 88 hours a week.

The recommendations of the Task Force were accepted by the Council of Review Committee Chairs, and in September 2010 the ACGME Board of Directors approved new rules that would go into effect July 1, 2011.

The patient safety community was disappointed. The reaction focused on duty hours. Most didn't believe the ACGME was making a commitment to ensure adequate supervision and a better learning environment.

In fact, the major thrust of the ACGME report was not about duty hours; it was about the learning environment. The Task Force was explicit: "The goal of the ACGME's new approach to duty hours is to foster a humanistic environment for graduate medical education that supports learning and the provision of excellent and safe patient care. The graduate medical education community has a moral responsibility to prepare residents to practice medicine outside the learning environment, where they will be unsupervised, must think independently, and must function when fatigued" [34].

"Paramount is an environment characterized by supervision customized to residents' level of competence, faculty modeling of fitness for duty, and the provision of high-quality care in a team setting and an institutional culture of safety." The new standards reflected this commitment.

The seriousness of the commitment of the ACGME to changing the learning environment was made clear by the significant expansion of its role. It would establish a new program of annual site visits of sponsoring institutions that would be separate from accreditation and would not focus just on duty hour compliance but also on supervision and the provision of a safe and effective environment for care and learning.

This was a big change, and it should have a major impact on residency training and patient safety. It is what Sidney Zion called for 25 years earlier.

The recommendation of the Duty Hours Task Force for evaluating the learning environment did not arise de novo. Ten years earlier there had been discussions at ACGME about how to improve the design of residency and fellowship programs through the use of a developmental framework and move the accreditation system to a focus on outcomes using a continuous quality improvement philosophy [37].

In 2009, ACGME CEO Tom Nasca convened a group of healthcare quality and patient safety experts, chaired by Carolyn Clancy, director of AHRQ, and Timothy Flynn, the chair of the ACGME Board of Directors, to make recommendations on how residency programs could be motivated to do a better job in training residents in patient safety.

One of the problems was that Graduate Medical Education programs were often managed at the department level, while quality and safety efforts were carried out at the hospital level from which the residents were not commonly included. How could they be integrated?

The group recommended that ACGME conduct an additional type of on-site visit, separate from and unrelated to accreditation visits. These visits would evaluate the learning environment, the residents' progress in achieving competencies, how they were integrated into the quality and safety activities of the hospital, and how programs were dealing with concerns about disparities and transitions in care.

CLER

To implement this ambitious program, Nasca brought Kevin Weiss, a member of the quality and safety workgroup and an immediate past CEO and president of the American Board of Medical Specialties into ACGME to develop the program. ACGME labeled it Clinical Learning Environment Review (CLER).

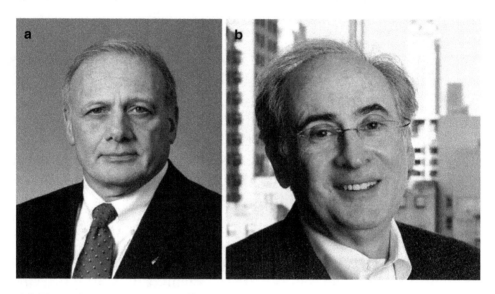

(**a**) Tom Nasca and (**b**) Kevin Weiss

The core of the CLER Program is a commitment to formative assessment and feedback regarding a residency training program's engagement in six focus areas: patient safety; health-care quality; care transitions; supervision; fatigue management, mitigation, and duty hours; and professionalism. The CLER Program required biannual formative assessment by each accredited sponsor of graduate medical education. It was designed to provide direct feedback to teaching hospitals and health-care organizations and to inform the ACGME accreditation process on issues in the six focus areas [38].

Training programs were now labeled Clinical Learning Environments (CLEs). Through periodic site visits that involve the program directors, residents, and the CEOs, the program aims to stimulate conversations and motivate CLEs to build upon their strengths and internally address opportunities for improvement.

Visits focus on six areas of concern: (1) the engagement and demonstration of meaningful participation of residents in the patient safety programs of the institution; (2) the engagement and demonstration of meaningful participation of residents in the institutional quality of care activities and participation in programs related to reduction of disparities in clinical care conducted by the institution; (3) the establishment and oversight of institutional supervision policies; (4) the effectiveness of institutional oversight of transitions of care; (5) the effectiveness of duty hours and fatigue mitigation policies; and (6) activities addressing the professionalism of the educational environment [39].

Milestones

In addition to the CLER program, ACGME established the milestone program. ACGME standards require residency and fellowship program directors to periodically assess each individual resident and fellow. These assessments use a variety of tools, including direct observations; global evaluation; audits and review of clinical performance data; multisource feedback from peers, nurses, patients, and family, simulation; self-assessment; and in-service training examinations [40].

ACGME requires semi-annual assessment of each resident and fellow on their progress in achieving *milestones* in the six domains of clinical competency that had been described as relevant for all medical practice by the ACGME and the ABMS in 1999. (See Chap. 20 for a discussion of the six competencies.)

Residency programs had for some time been required to configure curricula and evaluation processes in the framework of the six competencies under the Outcome Project, launched in 2001. Achieving the competencies was, in fact, the *purpose* of the programs. Under the ACGME, the training programs would ensure achievement of the six competencies. Certification programs, under the ABMS, would ensure that physicians maintained them.

Implementing outcome-based, i.e., competency-based, education into residency training was a big challenge for programs. Program directors and faculty had struggled since the launch of the Outcome Project to understand what competencies meant and what they looked like in practice [39]. They had different ideas of how to do it and different sets of skills for making the changes. There was wide variation between specialties and between programs within a specialty.

The concept of developmental milestones grew out of this need to move the outcomes project forward and deal with these variations. Milestones use narratives to describe the educational and professional trajectories of residents from the beginning of their education through the achievement of competency and the ability to enter into the unsupervised practice of medicine [40]. They define the stages in achieving competency for each of the six domains (Boxes 18.1 and 18.2).

Box 18.1 Milestone template

Milestone description: template

Level 1	Level 2	Level 3	Level 4	Level 5
What are the expectations for a beginning resident?	What are the milestones for a resident who has advanced over entry, but is performing at a lower level than expected at mid-residency?	What are the key developmental milestones mid-residency? What should they be able to do well in the realm of the specialty at this point?	What does a graduating resident look like? What additional knowledge, skills, and attitudes have they obtained? Are they ready for certification?	Stretch goals – exceeds expectations

Ref. [40]

Box 18.2 Milestones for systems-based practice 1: patient safety and quality improvement

SBP1: Patient safety and quality improvement

Level 1	Level 2	Level 3	Level 4	Level 5
Demonstrates knowledge of common patient safety events	Identifies system factors that lead to patient safety events	Participates in analysis of patient safety events (simulated or actual)	(simulated or actual)	Actively engages teams and processes to modify systems to prevent patient safety events
Demonstrates knowledge of how to report patient safety events	Reports patient safety events through institutional reporting systems (actual or simulated)	Participates in disclosure of patient safety events to patients and families (simulated or actual)	Discloses patient safety events to patients and families (simulated or actual)	Role models or mentors others in the disclosure of patient safety events
Demonstrates knowledge of basic quality improvement methodologies and metrics	Describes local quality improvement initiatives (e.g., community vaccination rate, infection rate, smoking cessation)	Participates in local quality improvement initiatives	Demonstrates the skills required to identify, develop, implement, and analyze a quality improvement project	Creates, implements, and assesses quality improvement initiatives at the institutional or community level

Ref. [40]

"Simply stated, the Milestones describe performance levels residents and fellows are expected to demonstrate for skills, knowledge, and behaviors in the six clinical competency domains. They lay out a framework of observable behaviors and other attributes associated with a resident's or fellow's development as a physician. The Milestones' primary purpose is to drive improvement in training programs and enhance the resident and fellow educational experience." [39]

Milestones were officially launched in 2013 in seven core specialties (emergency medicine, internal medicine, neurological surgery, orthopedic surgery, pediatrics, diagnostic radiology, and urology) as a component of the new accreditation system. The remaining core disciplines and the majority of subspecialties implemented the milestones a year later.

The CLER program and the Milestones have transformed residency training from an apprentice system—"do what I do"—measured by time served, into an educational system measured by competency achieved through planned experiences that include not only technical competency and knowledge, but experience in quality and safety and systems improvement.

Duty Hours

What happened about duty hours? Opposition to the 80-hour limit died a quiet death as evidence piled up against it. The ACGME funded two randomized trials that compared programs that strictly adhered to the rules to those with the flexible ones. The results showed that violations of 80-hour rules were linked to increased depression, suicide, and harm, such as needlestick injuries [25]. They also showed no differences in outcomes among surgery programs, leading to the conclusion that they should be bound by the same hour limits [41].

The other bit of evidence that the 80-hour limit was not harmful came from New York. The state had been strictly enforcing the 80-hour limit, with substantial fines, for a long time. No one could prove that physicians trained in New York were less competent. Skeptics began to come around. At the 2015 ACGME conference of Review Committees and others interested in graduate medical education, every medical organization agreed on the 80-hour limit. Shortly afterward it was adopted as a standard. The ACGME now cites programs if more than one resident in a program has violated the 80-hour limit.

Is the issue of duty hours settled, then? Hardly. Why is an 80-hour work week acceptable? Why is 13 hours a day, 6 days a week, with 1 weekend off a month considered humane given the damage it does to residents' well-being and family life? Talk about "normalizing deviance"!

Why do we turn a blind eye to the experience of the rest of the Western world—the EU limits that show competent and caring doctors can be trained in 48 hours a week? Forty-eight versus eighty! A world of difference. Could we train good—excellent—doctors in 48 hours a week, or at most 60? Of course we could.

They might even be better doctors. One of the major lessons in patient safety is that you can't expect health-care workers to care about patients' safety when you don't care about worker safety. Why do we think that treating doctors inhumanely will lead them to be kind and caring for their patients? Perhaps patients' complaints about how they are treated by their physician stem from how we treat the doctors during their formative training years.

Conclusion

What do we make of all this? The conflict over duty hours subsided with the "victory" of the 80-hour work week. On the other hand, the aggressive stance of the ACGME regarding the learning environment has been a welcome change and the CLER program has had an impact.

The implications for patient safety are also profound. A major stumbling block in advancing patient safety has been the lack of buy-in by most physicians; they don't "own" it. As Kevin Weiss points out, the profession doesn't "own" anything until it makes it an expectation of training and builds it into the training standards for the profession. That is where we agree on the definition of what the next generation must know and be able to do. Where we agree on who we are. The requirements for accreditation are therefore essential to how the profession is able to establish professional identity for all those who enter the profession (Kevin B. Weiss, MD, personal communication, May 20, 2020).

The groundwork was laid when the ABMS and ACGME agreed on the six domains of competency that included systems-based practice. The turning point was when ACGME expectations for training programs based on the six competencies became *requirements*. After evidence showed that programs were falling woefully short, the first CLER report outlined the needs for learning in quality and safety. These were later cut and pasted as requirements for accreditation.

Thanks to Tom Nasca and the ACGME, residency training has changed more in the past 20 years than in all of the previous 100. It is finally beginning to become more about education than service, about creating good physicians, not exploiting them. We now aspire to educate the whole physician, one who is skilled and expert, works well with others in teams, and communicates well with patients and colleagues.

The duty hours issue still needs work. We still have sleepy doctors. It's time to say good-bye to the 80-hour week and create a more humane environment. But we've made immense progress, and we are almost certainly turning out better doctors.

References

1. Lerner BH. A case that shook medicine: how one man's rage over his daughter's death sped reform of doctor training. The Washington Post. 2006; Lifestyle.
2. Sack K. Appeals court clears doctors who were censured in the Libby Zion case. The New York Times. 1991;B:2.
3. 2001 AAMC survey of housestaff stipends, senefits and funding. Washington, DC: AAMC; 2001.
4. New York State Department of Health's Ad Hoc Advisory Committee on Emergency Services. Supervision and residents' working conditions. New York; 1987.

5. New York Codes, Rules, and Regulations, Title 10 Section 405.4 Medical Staff (10 CRR-NY 405.4). In: New York State Department of Health, ed; 1988.
6. Lees DE. New York state regulations to be implemented. Anesth Patient Saf Found Newsl. 1988;3(3)
7. Accreditation. Accreditation Council for Graduate Medical Education (ACGME). https://www.acgme.org/What-We-Do/Accreditation. Accessed 6 June 2020.
8. Resident assessment: compliance with working hour and supervision requirements. New York: New York State Department of Health; 1998.
9. Health Care Reform Act of 2000, Bill No. A09093/S06187. In: New York State Assembly.
10. Gurjala A, Lurie P, Wolfe S. Petition to the occupational safety and health administration requesting that limits be placed on hours worked by medical residents (HRG Publication #1570). Public Citizen. https://www.citizen.org/article/petition-requesting-medical-residents-work-hour-limits/. Published April 30, 2001. Accessed 6 June 2020.
11. H.R.3236 – Patient and Physician Safety and Protection Act of 2001. In: House of Representatives 107th Congress 1st Session, ed: U.S. Congress.
12. Barnard A. Surgery residents' long hours draw warning for Yale. The Boston Globe. 2002;A1.
13. Philibert I, Friedmann P, Williams WT. Education AWGoRDHACfGM. New requirements for resident duty hours. JAMA. 2002;288(9):1112–4.
14. Daugherty SR, Baldwin JDC, Rowley BD. Learning, satisfaction, and mistreatment during medical internship: a national survey of working conditions. JAMA. 1998;279(15):1194–9.
15. Schwartz RJ, Dubrow TJ, Rosso RF, Williams RA, Butler JA, Wilson SE. Guidelines for surgical residents' working hours: intent vs reality. Arch Surg. 1992;127(7):778–83.
16. Report of the ACGME Work Group on Resident Duty Hours. Chicago: Accreditation Council for Graduate Medical Education; 2002.
17. Sleep-Deprived Doctors. The New York Times. June 14, 2002; Editorials/Letters: A36.
18. Gabehart RJ, Van Dongen HPA. Circadian rhythms in sleepiness, alertness, and performance. In: Kryger MH, Roth T, Dement WC, editors. Principles and practice of sleep medicine. 6th ed. Philadelphia: Elsevier; 2011. p. 388–95.
19. Dinges DF, Pack F, Williams K, et al. Cumulative sleepiness, mood disturbance, and psychomotor vigilance performance decrements during a week of sleep restricted to 4-5 hours per night. Sleep. 1997;20(4):267–77.
20. Dawson D, Reid K. Fatigue, alcohol and performance impairment. Nature. 1997;388(6639):235.

21. Gaba DM, Howard SK. Fatigue among clinicians and the safety of patients. N Engl J Med. 2002;347(16):1249–55.
22. Landrigan C, Rothschild J, Cronin J, et al. Effect of reducing interns' work hours on serious medical errors in intensie care units. N Engl J Med. 2004;351:1838–48.
23. Czeisler CA. Medical and genetic differences in the adverse impact of sleep loss on performance: ethical considerations for the medical profession. Trans Am Clin Climatol Assoc. 2009;120:249–85.
24. Weinger MB, Ancoli-Israel S. Sleep deprivation and clinical performance. JAMA. 2002;287(8):955–7.
25. Ayas NTB, Barger LK, Cade BE, Hashimoto DM, Rosner B, Cronin JW, Speizer FE, Czeisler CA. Extended work duration and the risk of self-reported percutaneous injuries in interns. JAMA. 2006;296(9):1055–62.
26. Barger L, Cade BE, Ayas NT, et al. Extended work shifts and the risk of motor vehicle crashes among interns. N Engl J Med. 2005;352:125–34.
27. Drazen JM, Epstein AM. Rethinking medical training--the critical work ahead. N Engl J Med. 2002;347(16):1271–2.
28. Stoddard JJ, Kindig DA, Libby D. Graduate medical education reform: service provision transition costs. JAMA. 1994;272(1):53–8.
29. Landrigan CPB, Barger LK, Cade BE, Ayas NT, Czeisler CA. Interns' compliance with accreditation council for graduate medical education work-hour limits. JAMA. 2006;296(9):1063–70.
30. Lockley S, Cronin JW, Evans EE, et al. Effect of reducing interns' weekly work hours on sleep and attentional failures. N Engl J Med. 2004;351:1829–37.
31. Levine AC, Adusumilli J, Landrigan CP. Effects of reducing or eliminating resident work shifts over 16 hours: a systematic review. Sleep. 2010;33(8):1043–53.
32. Reed DA, Fletcher KE, Arora VM. Systematic review: association of shift length, protected sleep time, and night float with patient care, residents' health, and education. Ann Intern Med. 2010;153(12):829–42.
33. Ulmer C, Wolman D, Johns M. Resident duty hours. Washington: The National Academies Press; 2009.
34. Nasca TJ, Day SH, Amis ES. The new recommendations on duty hours from the ACGME task force. N Engl J Med. 2010;363(2):e3.
35. Blum AB, Shea S, Czeisler C, Landrigan CP, Leape L. Implementing the 2009 Institute of Medicine recommendations on resident physician work hours, supervision, and safety. Nature Sci Sleep. 2011;3:47–85.
36. Blum AB, Raiszadeh F, Shea S, et al. US public opinion regarding proposed limits on resident physician work hours. BMC Med. 2010;8(33). Published online 2010 Jun 1. https://doi.org/10.1186/1741-7015-8-33.
37. Nasca TJ, Philibert I, Brigham T, Flynn TC. The next GME accreditation system — rationale and benefits. N Engl J Med. 2012;366(11):1051–6.
38. Clinical Learning Environment Review (CLER). Accreditation Council for Graduate Medical Education (ACGME). https://www.acgme.org/

What-We-Do/Initiatives/Clinical-Learning-Environment-Review-CLER. Accessed 6 June 2020.

39. Holmboe ES, Edgar L, Hamstra S. The milestones guidebook: ACGME; 2016.

40. Holmboe ES, Yamazaki K, Edgar L, et al. Reflections on the first 2 years of milestone implementation. J Grad Med Educ. 2015;7(3):506–11.

41. Rosen KA, Loveland AS, Romano SP, et al. Effects of resident duty hour reform on surgical and procedural patient safety indicators among hospitalized veterans health administration and medicare patients. Med Care. 2009;47(7):723–31.

19

Communication and Resolution of Errors

When patients are harmed by their treatment, they want three things from their doctor: they want the doctor to tell them what happened, say they are sorry, and tell them what will be done to keep it from happening to someone else. "What happened" is an acknowledgment that something went wrong, followed by an explanation of why it happened, and some guidance on what the future holds. If they have additional medical expenses or a disability, they also want compensation. Sadly, none of this happens most of the time [1].

The psychological harm following injury can be devastating. Feelings of fear, betrayal, anxiety about the future, and anger are common. Yet this aspect of patient safety was scarcely mentioned in the medical literature or in discussions prior to the patient safety movement. An exception was the work of Charles Vincent, who wrote in 1994 about why patients sue doctors. He described the mix of feelings of fear, loss of trust, and not knowing what happened [2]. In fact, for the patient the psychological trauma often exceeds the physical. It is those feelings, not pain or a long convalescence, that they remember years later.

In 2003, Gallagher conducted focus groups of patients to learn about their experiences and opinions about disclosure. They corroborated Vincent's findings. He found that becoming aware of an error in their care made patients "sad, anxious, depressed, or traumatized." Patients feared additional errors, were angry that their recovery had been prolonged, and were frustrated that the error was preventable

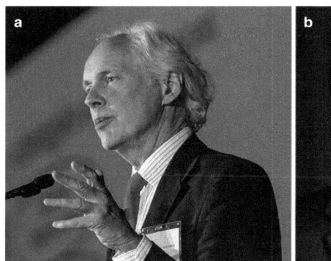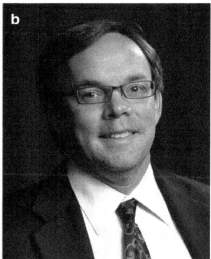

(a) Charles Vincent and (b) Tom Gallagher.

[3]. Patients said they would be less upset if the doctor disclosed the error compassionately and apologized.

While medicine seemed to pay little attention to patients' feelings, there was a continuing thread in the medical literature over the years about the effects that errors had on the physician. Perhaps the most powerful was by David Hilfiker, who in 1984 wrote a poignant piece in the New England Journal of Medicine, "Facing Our Mistakes," that described his personal anguish dealing with his patients and his own feelings after harming a patient by his error [4]. In 1985 and in 1988, Vincent reported on the devastating effect that making an error has on physicians [5]. In 1991, Albert Wu wrote of the problems house officers had in talking about mistakes and coined the term "second victim," [6] and in 1992, Christensen wrote of the profound effects of their errors on physicians [7].

The second victim's emotional state is potentially harmful to the patient as well. It clouds the physician's judgment, increasing the risk of committing a second error. It makes empathetic communication difficult at just the time when it is most important.

But neither of these powerful forces—the devastating effects of unexpected harm on patients and on their physicians—was much in the discussion about communicating with patients after an error, either before or after the IOM report. Instead, the arguments tended to be framed in terms of duty: honest disclosure is the "right thing to do," it is the "ethical" thing to do, "we have a professional obligation to be honest with our patients," etc.

Not that it is the kind thing to do, the healing thing to do, the human thing to do. Nor that effective and empathetic communication is the *necessary* thing to do, that it is the appropriate medical *treatment*—effective and science-based—for this second injury we had caused.

And, although principles were declared and practices for disclosure were recommended by elite medical organizations, including the AMA and the Joint Commission, they lacked force; open and honest communication following medical harm remained the exception, not the rule.

As noted previously, the most powerful—and most remembered—event at the very first patient safety meeting, the 1996 Annenberg Conference, was the presentation of the case of Ben Kolb, a boy who died from a medication mix-up in the operating room. What was memorable to the audience was that the hospital was open and transparent about it from the beginning, admitting error and apologizing. It was memorable because it was so rare. Few medical people in the audience thought such a case would be handled that way in their institution.

The very word used to describe these conversations, *disclosure*, tells much about the problem. It clearly implies ownership and choice. Information about the details of what happened and possible wrongdoing is deemed to belong to the physician, not the patient; it is the physician's choice whether, and how much of, this secret information should be *disclosed* to the patient. The high-flown rhetoric about honesty, honor, and professionalism and the duty to disclose reinforce the concept that the information belongs to the physician.

Not surprisingly, this idea is totally rejected by patient advocate groups, who reasonably ask, "Whose body is it anyway?"

Important as these concerns are, they have traditionally had little bearing on what actually happens. Rationality, empathy, logic, duty, and, sadly, even ethics play a distant second fiddle to the real reasons that doctors are not open and honest with their patients: shame and fear. Shame silences doctors, but fear drives the debate: the fear of being sued for malpractice.

Malpractice

It is not an irrational fear. The conventional wisdom for decades was that you made mistakes because you weren't careful enough. It was your fault, doctor. This thinking was reinforced by the lawyers and the courts, who took the position that an error is *by definition* a failure to meet the standard of care; failure to meet the standard of care in turn is the definition of negligence, of malpractice.

This is not true, of course. Making a mistake is not negligence, it is part of normal human behavior. That is the point of the patient safety movement. But the lawyers didn't believe that. They would have us believe that if you admit to making a mistake, or even if you acknowledge that something went wrong, you are asking to be sued for malpractice.

Defense lawyers—those who worked for hospitals and doctors— saw their responsibility as protecting the doctor or hospital from being sued regardless of whether there was negligence. The way they sought to do that was to get the doctors to "stonewall" from the beginning: tell the patient nothing, don't admit error, and, by all means, never apologize. Liability insurers, anxious to minimize losses, reinforced this message. Many even told physicians that if they admitted error, their insurance would not cover them.

Doctors went along. Admitting error, especially an error that has hurt your patient who trusted you, is painfully difficult. Being told by an authority not to admit anything gave them cover for not doing something they really didn't want to do. If the lawyers recommended it, then perhaps it was all right, even though it did violate their code of professionalism and even though deep down they knew it was wrong.

A word about malpractice suits. When a claim is filed, a protracted period of several years or more follows during which the physician must go back over the case in minute detail in multiple interviews with lawyers and depositions from the opposing side, while constantly dreading the trial itself. Often, the physician does not believe he did anything wrong. In fact, he may not even have made a mistake, or if he did, it was no worse than anyone else's, and he certainly didn't intend harm. But intent has nothing to do with it in tort law. (If the injury were intended, it would be criminal assault.)

Nor does the fact that we now know that almost all errors result from multiple systemic factors. In addition, in the USA, the focus of medical liability has long been on the physician, so that is who insurance policies cover. That is where the money is, so that is who the malpractice lawyer goes after. Medical negligence is about the individual not meeting the standard of care, defined as "what a reasonably prudent specialist should do under the same or similar circumstances."

Although safety experts hold that in most cases it is the hospital that should be held liable since it is responsible for the systems that fail and cause harm, that is a relatively new concept and still not widely accepted. Moreover, most hospitals were, until recently, charitable organizations for which states have traditionally provided immunity or very limited liability.

In a malpractice trial, the plaintiff's lawyer's task is to convince the jury not only that the doctor's action harmed the patient, but that the physician was careless, even reckless. The trial is an exercise in public humiliation, drawn out over a week or more: not only did the doctor do a bad thing, he or she is a bad person. No wonder doctors dread it and do whatever they can to avoid it.

Medicine is the only profession consistently subjected to this type of humiliation. Not just a few, but *most* physicians are sued at least once in their professional career, and some, especially those in the high-risk specialties such as vascular surgery and neurosurgery, are sued multiple times. The average neurosurgeon is said to spend 25% of their time in malpractice litigation.

In addition to fear of being sued for malpractice, doctors had other reasons to perpetuate a "conspiracy of silence." Admitting a mistake, most believed, would undermine their patient's trust of the physician. Colleagues would think less of them. Both their professional and their public reputations would be tarnished, perhaps irrevocably damaged. Referring relationships might be diminished and their income suffer.

But the most powerful deterrent to open communication is shame. The roots are deep within the physician's psyche, the product of the high-achieving personalities that are attracted to medicine. It is enhanced by an educational system that sets perfect performance as the standard and of a cultural environment that reinforces it. Admitting—to yourself or to others—that you have made a serious error is admitting that you have failed to live up to your own standard of perfect performance to prevent harm to your patient.

For the physician, making a serious error is not just a practice failure, it is a character failure. The shame can be overwhelming. With their self-esteem so at risk, it is not surprising that physicians develop defense mechanisms, such as denial that an error occurred or displacement of blame to an underling. Failing that, they desperately want to keep it a secret.

When I first began to comprehend the power of approaching medical errors as systems failures in the early 1990s, it seemed to me that a systems approach would not only reduce harm to patients, it would immensely benefit physicians. If doctors bought into the concept that errors are caused by systems failures, not personal failures, the burden of shame and guilt would be lifted from their shoulders, enabling them to be open and honest with their patients. While this is attractive in theory, in practice it has yet to happen on any significant scale.

Not only have malpractice concerns totally dominated the thinking about disclosure, some have argued that full disclosure would significantly *increase* the number of liability suits and total costs. Their reasoning held that if all patients were informed about an error, a significant number of patients who otherwise would not have known would be added to the pool of patients who might sue [8].

The Contrarians

The first chink in the wall of silence appeared in 1999, about the time *To Err Is Human* came out. Steve Kraman and Ginny Hamm published the experience from the Veterans Administration Hospital in Lexington, Kentucky, which in 1987 had instituted a policy of full disclosure and compensation following harm from a negligent medical error. A review of 88 cases from 1990 to 1996 revealed total hospital annual payments were less than half the rate in previous years [9].

Unfortunately, although the entire VHA adopted a disclosure policy that patients be informed of unintended outcomes, it did not extend Kraman's program to the entire system. VHA continued the practice of not explaining why things went wrong and not apologizing.

In Colorado, COPIC, the state's largest liability insurer, in 2000 developed the "3Rs" (recognize, respond, resolve) program of "no-fault" compensation to forestall litigation. It provides patients up to $30,000 for out-of-pocket health-care expenses and lost work time. They do not offer explanations or apologies and make the offer only in cases where the patient has not filed a claim. It is a structured service recovery operation, in effect an expansion of long-standing insurance practices aimed at loss control. It has been effective in reducing litigation, however. In one reported 5-year period, it handled over 3000 cases and reduced payouts and lawsuits dramatically [10, 11].

The real breakthrough came a few years later when Rick Boothman, Chief Risk Officer of University of Michigan Health System, reported their experience with a program he instituted in 2001 of responding to claims by admitting fault and offering compensation if internal investigation revealed "that the injury resulted from care that fell below expectations." The program was not limited to disclosure but linked to quality and safety efforts and expanded to identify injuries by various means. If an error was found, fault was admitted, and compensation was given for lifelong medical expenses, lost wages, and other costs—all without the patient needing to file a claim.

Analysis of results over a 5-year period following full implementation of the program showed a reduction of suits by 65% and decreases in legal costs and payouts to patients by more than 50% each. Total liability costs per year dropped from $3 million to $1 million [12].

Boothman emphasizes that the more important impact was on the culture. Full disclosure after unplanned clinical outcomes became the leading edge of changing the culture within the organization to increase transparency. Transparency is the key to a learning culture that facilitates internal reporting of adverse events and dealing with disruptive behavior and other performance problems. Full and open case investigations are necessary if we are to learn from our mistakes and advance the systems thinking that safety requires [13]. Boothman observed that in those organizations in which open disclosure failed, leadership did not connect it to their core mission and did not actively support adoption against the skeptics [13].

So, the arguments against full disclosure and apology were wrong: patients weren't more likely to sue, they were *less* likely to sue. And the costs went down not up. Trust depends on honesty, so it is not surprising that patients' trust in their physicians is enhanced, not diminished, by the doctor's forthright admission of failure and taking responsibility for it. Being honest is not only the morally and ethically right thing to do, it is the smart thing to do.

An interesting sidebar: at a lawyers' conference on malpractice that I attended about this time, a prominent Houston plaintiff's lawyer boasted about the number of patients who came to him to sue their doctor and then said, "Ninety percent of them wouldn't be there if the doctor had just told them what happened and said he was sorry!"

Physicians agreed in principle but had trouble doing it. They were cautious about how much to tell patients and believed that apology would be used as evidence of liability. They chose their words carefully, sometimes acknowledging the harm but not disclosing the error, why it happened, or what would be done to prevent recurrences. They were unlikely to discuss minor errors or near misses [3].

But things were beginning to change. At about this time, Gallagher issued a call for action by physicians, hospitals, certifying boards, accrediting bodies, medical societies, and medical educators to develop policies for disclosure, train physicians in communication, and provide support for patients and doctors [14].

Also in 2005, two senators, Hillary Clinton and Barack Obama, introduced the National Medical Error Disclosure and Compensation (MEDiC) Act that emphasized open disclosure, apology, early compensation, and analysis of the event. It was offered as a means of addressing both patient safety and the problems with the liability system. Although it never passed, it put the issue on the national agenda [15].

Doing It Right

Responding appropriately after a serious harmful event is not as simple as it may seem to those who have never had to do it. It is a highly emotionally charged moment for the patient and the physician. The patient is frightened, and if the harm resulted from an error the physician may be overwhelmed with feelings of shame and guilt. It is not a situation conducive to thoughtful supportive communication. The patient needs immediate reassurance from their doctor, primarily that they will be all right, and an explanation of what happened, but the initial talk is not the time to speculate on causes or details of what happened. They need to know *what* happened, not yet *why* it happened.

The physician should be honest and transparent, acknowledge that something has gone wrong, and explain what happened and what is being done to counter its effects. They should express regret—"I'm sorry this happened to you"—but avoid commenting on the cause of the event or apologizing, because investigation may reveal information that contradicts the initial assumptions of culpability. The patient should be told that an investigation will be carried out and the results will be given to them as soon as it is completed.

If investigation reveals that the injury was caused by an error, the physician needs to apologize. As the person responsible for the patient's care, the doctor in charge is the one to apologize, even if the error was made by a resident, a nurse, the pathologist, or someone else. The patient looks to their personal physician to make sure care is safe. The other person should accompany the physician if appropriate.

The CEO or other high-ranking administrator should also be there to apologize for the failure of the hospital's systems to prevent the injury. Although the patient understandably holds the person who made the error responsible, since errors result from systems failures, it is important for the patient to hear that from someone other than the physician, from whom it would seem self-serving.

A meaningful apology must include three elements: remorse, accountability, and amends. The physician must communicate their genuine deep feelings of sorrow, "I feel terrible about what happened." They must also take responsibility, "We let you down, it should not have occurred." The exact words are not critical, but it must come from the heart. Mere words, however "correct," will not do.

Meaningful apology also includes making every possible effort to make up for the injury. This means financial compensation for all expenses related to the injury, present and future. In addition to medical expenses, these include lost wages, extra household costs, and long-term effects of disability. Without restitution, apology is a gesture.

These are difficult conversations, and they will not occur unless there is serious advance planning. Physicians need to be trained in disclosure—which is not easy since it is so painful for them—and they need support in the moment. They need help in apologizing. Fortunately, for most physicians these conversations occur rarely, but that means they need coaching and support when they do.

This is where the hospital comes in. Ideally, the risk management department has shifted its focus from limiting liability to limiting (emotional) harm to both the patient and the doctor and is integrated with the quality and safety programs and nursing and physician administration. If not, a team needs to be developed in the quality and safety group. A training program is essential for teaching physicians how to communicate in this difficult situation, and it should be required for all physicians, who will find it difficult and painful.

Hospitals must also have support systems for both the patient and the doctor, as well as the nurse and support staff. Open, honest disclosure diminishes the patient's fears and anxiety, but it doesn't take it away. The patient needs comforting and understanding. So does the doctor. Even if they succeed at communicating with the patient after a serious event as a result of their training and excellent coaching, the shame and guilt don't go away. A colleague's arm around the shoulder and a reassuring word can go a long way, but more is needed. A system is needed to make sure both patients and doctors get emotional support in these first traumatic days.

Some years ago, a seriously injured patient in Boston, Linda Kenney, began to create that system. From her own experience, Linda recognized that the best support would come from a peer – someone who had been through a similar experience. With Rick VanPelt, the anesthesiologist involved in her episode, she founded Medically Induced Trauma Support Services (MITSS) to help hospitals develop peer support systems both for patients and families and for clinicians and staff. Thousands of people have been trained by this program, which is now a division of the Betsy Lehman Center for Patient Safety [16] .

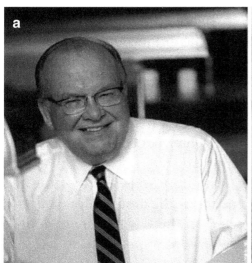 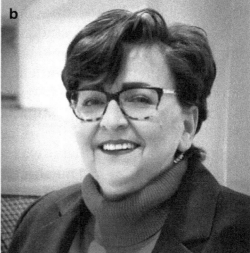

(**a**) Rick Boothman and (**b**) Linda Kenney.

Truly effective support requires changing the institution's culture away from punishment to learning—the basic challenge of the safety movement. Away from the hushed comment and pointed fingers, from "Isn't it too bad about Charlie" or "We all make mistakes" to a culture that really does look at an adverse event as a "treasure," an opportunity to learn how the system failed—and fixes it. A culture that recognizes that, with rare exceptions, the physician is not the cause of the error but the victim of it.

When Things Go Wrong—The Disclosure Project

Gallagher's work and Kraman's and Boothman's experiences changed the discussion in the patient safety world but seemed to have little impact on the practice in hospitals. Most of the principle players: hospitals, doctors, defense lawyers, and liability insurers were skeptical. The VA and Michigan were "different." Too risky to take a chance— although, of course, it was "the right thing to do."

Harvard hospitals were no exception. The ones that I was close to were not changing their policies or practices. CRICO, the Harvard hospitals' umbrella liability insurance company that funded our early error research, was proud of its record defending doctors and saw no need to change. Despite my entreaties and those of others, they and the hospitals were loath to take a chance. They gave lip service to full disclosure but did little to facilitate it. I stewed about this for some time. I would teach my students about the importance of honesty, communication, and apology, but I knew it wasn't happening.

How to get it moving? Perhaps if it were possible to get the leadership of all of the Harvard hospitals to agree on a uniform policy of full disclosure, apology, and restitution, it would stimulate their staff to actually do it. And if Harvard hospitals had success, perhaps that might persuade others that it was feasible and safe.

To see if this idea had any traction, I ran it by some of my frontline colleagues and friends: the safety leaders at the five major Harvard teaching hospitals. I asked them whether they were interested in exploring the issues about disclosure and apology. All responded enthusiastically.

The first meeting of what became the Disclosure Working Group was on May 10, 2004. Quality and safety leaders from the five hospitals were joined by two representatives from the Risk Management Foundation (RMF) of CRICO, and one from the Institute for Healthcare Improvement (IHI):

- *Janet Barnes*, nurse and risk manager at Brigham and Women's Hospital (BWH)
- *Maureen Connor*, risk manager at Dana-Farber Cancer Institute (DFCI)
- *Connie Crowley-Ganser*, vice president for quality at Boston Children's Hospital
- *Frank Federico*, pharmacist and quality leader at IHI
- *Bob Hanscom* and *Luke Sato* from CRICO/RMF
- *Cy Hopkins*, a quality and safety leader at Massachusetts General Hospital
- *Hans Kim*, quality specialist at Beth Israel Deaconess Medical Center

Review of their current institutional policies revealed that only three of the five hospitals had a written disclosure policy, and only one had a training program for physicians regarding disclosure. Clearly, we had work to do. Perhaps if we could spell out in detail what was needed and show how to do it, we would get buy-in.

At the second meeting a month later, we were joined by three new members, all physicians, Arnold Freedman, from DFCI, David Roberson from Children's, and Rick Van Pelt from BWH. John Ryan, the key CRICO/RMF lawyer, would join us at the next meeting. At this meeting, we made an important decision: in keeping with the systems concept, the policy should not focus on errors, but on adverse events.

At the July meeting, we made an even more important decision. Rather than limit our efforts to disclosure policy, we would craft a comprehensive document that addressed all aspects of responding to unanticipated events. No such statement existed; there were major assertions about disclosure (ASHRM, Minnesota Children's Hospital, etc.), and papers written about supporting patients and physicians, but no statements, policies, or recommendations that embraced all of the issues. Such a statement could have a major educational impact within our institutions at all levels. Much of the information and the rationale behind it would be new for many physicians.

The organizing principle, setting the "tone" of the statement, would be, "What is the right thing to do?" We defined the "right thing" as the institution taking responsibility to make things right by being open, informative, supportive, and restorative. We would try to break the mold of hospitals and doctors thinking about what is in their best interest to what is in the best interest of the patient.

We also agreed that the document needed to start off with the moral/ conceptual justification for this work. We are talking about much more than just disclosure or dealing with malpractice or the "business case." It is about hospitals meeting their obligation to respect patient's integrity, be sensitive to their needs, and earn their trust. This is the "do the right thing" part. Something like, "We hold these truths to be self-evident, that all patients are entitled to ... " (though not quite so grand—nor stolen!).

A bit late, but fortunately not too late, we suddenly realized that our group was missing the key stakeholder: the patient! To our great good fortune, Mary Dana Gershanoff and Gary Jernegan, co-chairs of the Dana-Farber Pediatric Patient & Family Advisory Council, were pleased to join us. When I told Tom Delbanco, an old friend and nationally respected physician patient advocate at BIDMC, about what we were doing, he expressed strong interest, so we asked him to join us as well. I was delighted, for his contributions were bound to be significant.

By March, we had a consensus document that we were happy with. We framed it in three parts: The Patient and Family Experience, The Caregiver Experience, and Management of the Event, with chapters on relevant issues. Each topic was organized into three sections: what should be done, why (the reasoning and evidence), and the specific recommendations. Following Tom Delbanco's recommendation, we titled it *When Things Go Wrong* [17].

When Things Go Wrong

The Patient and Family Experience

Three issues were addressed: communicating with the patient, support of the patient and family, and follow-up care of the patient and family.

The initial communication should occur promptly, within 24 hours. Patients have a right to be fully and promptly informed of any incident as soon as it is recognized. The physician responsible for the patient's care should acknowledge the event, take responsibility for it, express regret, and explain what happened. When results of the investigation are available, they should be communicated by the responsible physician and involve the CEO or CMO in serious cases. If an error was found, the physician apologizes.

Support of the patient and family addresses their psychological, social, and financial needs. Patients should be asked about their feelings, provided with psychological support, and given attention to their continuing medical care. Immediate financial assistance should be given if needed. Hospitals should consider paying for all future expenses due to permanent disability and continuing medical treatment.

Follow-up care after discharge from the hospital requires the care team to provide continuing psychological and social support by maintaining communication through scheduled follow-up visits and telephone calls.

The Caregiver Experience

Like patients and families, caregivers are significantly impacted, emotionally and functionally, following an adverse event. They need support to recover and to communicate appropriately with the injured patient. Hospitals need to have training programs in communication with patients when things go wrong, and how to deal with their own feelings. They also need "just in time" coaching when events occur and training in supporting colleagues when in need.

Management of the Event

The hospital needs to have an incident policy that sets expectations and provides guidance for the staff to improve patient safety by learning from adverse events and changing systems.

The *elements* of the policy are a commitment to open and honest communication, provision of just-in-time guidance, education of caregivers in empathetic communicating, provision of emotional support, and systems of documentation and reporting.

The *initial response* is first to stabilize the patient and eliminate any remaining threat, to secure implicated drugs and equipment, and to provide a substitute provider if needed. The care team must be promptly briefed to ensure consistent communication with the patient and family. The person to communicate with the patient and family is decided upon. An investigation should be done quickly while memories are fresh. The event is reported to the appropriate hospital authority.

Analysis of the event is essential for several reasons: to prevent, if possible, a recurrence in a future patient, to satisfy the patient's right to know what the causes were and what is being done to remedy them, and to disseminate the learnings to other health-care organizations. Analyses should be multidisciplinary and nonjudgmental. The objective is to uncover the multiple factors that contributed to the event and, where possible, develop systems changes to make it less likely that the event will recur.

Documentation of the event is essential, as is *reporting*. The reporting policy should define the process for responding, identify who is to be notified, how, and by whom. Reporting must be safe for the caregiver and should lead to investigation and corrective action. When required, file reports with regulators.

We were pleased with our product. Nothing like this had been done before. We hoped it would motivate all of the Harvard hospitals, and others, to make major changes in how they handle patient harms. We made it clear up front that this was a call to action. Now to find out if anyone would respond to the call!

Getting Support

I went on a major selling job. RMF arranged a meeting with the Chief Medical Officers of all 14 Harvard-affiliated hospitals. I asked them to read the draft; discuss it with their local physicians, nurses, administrative leaders, and hospital counsel; and circulate it widely among staff. We asked them to tell us if this was an appropriate approach and to tell us how to make it better—within a month. They did—and we received a deluge of comments from many people in many of the hospitals. We were pleased that all were supportive of the effort, and we got a lot of good advice. This was the first step in building stakeholder support.

John Ryan, our legal representative from RMF, arranged for me to meet with the risk management lawyers from the major hospitals to get their input. At the meeting, I was pleased, and frankly a bit surprised, to find they had no problems with what we had written. That was a good sign!

However, they did have a concern that some doctors might apologize right away for something that was found on investigation to not be due to an error. Coming back to the patient later with a different story would be difficult. We changed the document to emphasize that the initial communication should be an expression of regret about the event. Apologizing would take place later if appropriate.

The committee member from each institution and I then met with all of the hospital CEOs and their key leaders, such as the CMO, CNO, and COO to discuss the paper and ask for their endorsement. We found them overall quite receptive. The CEOs of two of them, BWH and Children's Hospital sent me letters of support.

In July, an unfortunate thing happened. Liz Kowalczyk, a health reporter for the Boston Globe contacted me. She got wind of our project—hardly a surprise, since by now probably over 100 people had seen the draft—but she had not seen the draft. I told her that we would welcome an article on the final version, after the hospitals had approved it, but because of the sensitivity of the subject, they would have a negative reaction to anything coming out before all issues had been settled. It would make it harder to get them to sign on. I asked her to hold off for now. Despite that, she went ahead and published a substantial article on July 24.

As predicted, there were some strong reactions—particularly the MGH. Their CEO, Peter Slavin, was furious. I met with him and assured him that we had released no information and would not until everyone was signed on.

By September, we had incorporated many suggestions and had the revised, final version of the report. I then sent it to the CEOs with the request that "your institution endorse the principles and concepts in the document and commit to implementing them in your hospital." Recognizing that this would require approval at various levels, from medical executive committee to the Trustees, we asked for a response by December 1.

By November 15, we had a letter of endorsement signed by all seven of the Partners hospitals' CMOs! By mid-December, we knew we would get letters from all the rest, so we made plans to publish in the spring.

After getting the endorsement from the hospitals, I went to Harvard Medical School to see if we could also get them to endorse it and be the organization to publish it. I thought the combination would be very powerful—a statement coming from the school and all of its teaching hospitals.

They requested I provide letters from all of the hospital CMOs, which was easily done, and present it to the Academic Council. The meeting went well, there were no difficult questions, and I left thinking they were supportive. In the end, however, they decided not to endorse it. Having "jumped through all the hoops," I was very disappointed. It was yet another example of how difficult it is to navigate the political aspects of this sensitive subject.

Fortunately, their refusal did not hold us back nor have any long-term impact. Paula Griswold of the Massachusetts Coalition for the Prevention of Medical Errors Coalition was delighted to publish it. RMF agreed to pay for printing and mailing costs.

When the printed copies arrived, I went for maximum distribution. Copies were sent to the leaders of all of the hospitals, members of the Coalition, CRICO/RMF, IHI, NPSF, BCBS, as well as the head of every national organization with a stake in patient safety (AMA, ANA, AONE, Leapfrog, CAPS, advocacy groups, etc.) and to every person I knew in patient safety anywhere in the world.

It was well received. As we hoped, this comprehensive statement by an authoritative source gave those working in patient safety what they needed to start making disclosure and apology work in their hospitals. We hoped we had kick-started the process. Later feedback and citations in fact did indicate that it was widely disseminated and had significant influence.

National Progress in Communication and Resolution

While we were working to move communication and resolution ahead, the National Quality Forum (NQF) also had a committee working on it, although none of us were aware of it. Eight months after we published our report, the NQF issued a new Safe Practice on disclosure. The key elements were that the patient should be provided the facts about the event: whether there was an error and the results of event analysis, the physician should express regret and give formal apology if the outcome was caused by error or system failure. Institutions were to integrate disclosure, patient-safety, and risk-management activities and establish a support system with coaching and emotional support for patients and staff [18].

The NQF action changed the ballgame. The NQF cannot require any institution to implement its Safe Practices, but it is the respected source that regulators and overseers, such as the Joint Commission [19], AHRQ, and the Center for Medicare and Medicaid Services look to for establishing standards. Activity picked up.

In 2007, Stanford University Medical Network launched a claims management process called Process for Early Assessment, Resolution and Learning (PEARL). Although, like COPIC, it was not a full program that included apology and appropriate compensation for all injured patients, it did reduce suits and costs. They reported that in the first 3.5 years after implementation, claim frequency dropped 36%, with a cost savings of $3.2 million per fiscal year.

At the University of Illinois Medical Center at Chicago (UIMCC), Tim McDonald and David Mayer developed the "Seven Pillars" program derived from work done at Michigan to integrate communication with system improvement [20]. Mayer was Associate Dean for Education who had a deep interest in patient safety. In 2005 he started the Academy for Emerging Leaders in Patient Safety, a week-long program on patient safety at Telluride for medical students. There were 20 students. The program has since been expanded to include residents and is now given in four locations to over 150 a year.

In the Seven Pillars program, quality improvement efforts were directed to define or improve systems for all seven stages of the process: reporting, investigation, communication and disclosure, apology and remediation, system improvement, data tracking and analysis, and education and training.

They later reported that from 2002 to 2013, the intervention at UIMCC nearly doubled the number of incident reports, reduced the number of claims by 42%, reduced legal fees and costs by 51%, and reduced the number of lawsuits by 47% [21, 22].

In 2009, at the direction of President Obama, the US Department of Health and Human Services authorized AHRQ to launch a demonstration project on communication and resolution programs under its $23 million Patient Safety and Medical Liability grant. UIMCC and the University of Washington (UW) were among four health systems piloting chosen. UIMCC's demonstration project demonstrated that it was possible to package training and tools to disseminate the Seven Pillars approach to DRP to community hospitals settings. The UW intervention trained 1300 health-care providers in teaching skills in disclosure and apology [22].

But the full application of Boothman's work did not take off until Alan Woodward, an emergency physician and past president of Massachusetts Medical Society who was passionate about medical liability reform, and Kenneth Sands, chief quality officer of Beth Israel Deaconess Medical Center, developed a plan for getting widespread adoption of programs by involving all stakeholders.

They obtained a 1-year planning grant from AHRQ to create a roadmap for implementing a statewide Communication and Resolution Program (CRP) model. They interviewed dozens of key stakeholders in the medical liability arena and identified 12 significant obstacles to implementation and developed strategies to overcome each. The roadmap provided a guide for action [23].

Woodward then did something quite remarkable to assure success: he brought the lawyers on board. He persuaded the Massachusetts Bar Association and the Massachusetts Academy of Trial attorneys to join the Massachusetts Medical Society to promote CRP programs statewide. Not just to participate but to join in leading the new effort. This was not to be just a doctors' patient safety project.

Their first task was to create a more supportive legal environment. They developed consensus language for legislation that mandated sharing of all pertinent medical records, a 6 month pre-litigation resolution period, strong apology protections, and the obligation of hospitals to disclose any significant adverse outcome [24]. Given the support of the key parties, the legislature accepted their language without change as part of the 2012 comprehensive medical reform act, setting the stage for moving ahead with the new approach.

To implement the roadmap, the group formed the Massachusetts Alliance for Communication and Resolution following Medical Injury (MACRMI) with representation from statewide organizations with a stake in the medical liability process: physicians, hospitals, patient advocates, insurers, and attorneys.

MACRMI's goal was to develop, implement, and pilot a rigorous Communication, Apology, and Resolution Program (which it calls CARe), collect comprehensive data to assess its impact, and assist its dissemination. Modeled after the University of Michigan Health System's program, CARe promotes early resolution in cases of avoidable medical injury. When unanticipated adverse outcomes occur, patients and their families are provided full explanation of what happened, what it means for the patient medically, what will be done to prevent the error from happening again, and, where appropriate, a sincere apology and adequate and an offer of fair and timely compensation.

To achieve this goal, MACRMI developed an implementation guide with comprehensive resources, including best practices, algorithms, policies and procedures, teaching materials, and tracking tools (all available free on their website: www.macrmi.info). It then tested CARe and the toolkit in a pilot program in 6 hospitals over 3 years, collecting settlement data on nearly 1000 cases as well as patient experience and provider satisfaction survey information.

Data from the study showed that claims and costs did not increase, and more patients were compensated. The median compensation for these cases was $75,000, a number too low for a typical plaintiff's attorney to take the case. Of cases that reached the resolution stage, 41% gave rise to a safety measure that was or was likely to be implemented by the hospital. These included new labeling for high-risk medications, color-coded socks for patients at risk for falls, and a multidisciplinary checklist for breech deliveries [25, 26].

As a result of MACRMI's efforts, 12 health-care institutions in Massachusetts are now using CARe, and a number of others are moving toward it. In addition, several entities in other states are in the process of implementing programs [27].

But the impact of MACRMI is much greater than the early adoption numbers signify. What we are witnessing is the beginning of a culture change in the way we think about and respond to those we harm. A change in thinking not just in a group of hospitals and a physicians' group and a carrier, but in the governor's office, in the legislature, in the plaintiff's bar, in the defense bar and even in the courts. Patient safety—their welfare—and honesty are what CRP programs are about, not reducing losses in malpractice suits.

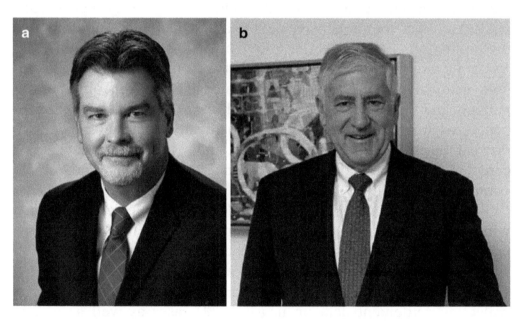

(**a**) David Mayer and (**b**) Alan Woodward.

From the experience of those in Massachusetts, Michigan, Washington, and others around the country, AHRQ developed the CANDOR (Communication and Optimal Resolution) initiative to proactively engage health-care providers, patients, and their family in preventable harm communications. It combines early event reporting, analysis, prompt, supportive and compassionate ongoing communication to the patient, fast, fair resolution where warranted, and applying lessons learned to change systems [28, 29].

AHRQ developed a CANDOR toolkit with input from those facilities awarded grants and other experts to help hospitals implement CRPs quickly and promoted its adoption. Several large health-care systems, including CentraCare and MedStar Health, have made commitments to its implementation, and the Medical Professional Liability Association and the Doctors Company have given it strong support [30].

Conclusion

The extensive activity on all fronts over the past two decades has dramatically changed the landscape for communication and resolution programs, increasing awareness of the urgency for change and providing an array of mechanisms to help health-care organizations implement new systems and provide the training and support that are needed.

But the challenges are immense. Implementing an effective system of communication, apology, and resolution is the cutting edge of the larger issue of transparency. Openness and honesty in communicating with patients is difficult in an institution that is not transparent in other ways, such as freedom to discuss errors and a willingness to go public with its mistakes. Creating transparency requires strong leadership.

CRP is also about another crucial aspect of a safety culture that is too often overlooked in the emphasis on reducing blame: accountability. The mindset of doctors and hospital leaders has to change to putting accountability ahead of fears of litigation and loss of reputation. To do this, strong leadership is required. CEOs have to stand up to the lawyers and insurers and insist they play their roles in that mission.

Even with strong leadership and a skilled team, teaching physicians to communicate effectively and empathetically after a serious preventable event is difficult. Unfortunately, lip service to CRP often outstrips true implementation. Needing to fulfill oversight demands, some hospitals initiate program improvements that focus selectively on claims resolution rather than on comprehensive programs of full communication, apology, and restitution that prioritize patient support and opportunities for improving quality and safety. While some patients are helped, many are not, and there is little learning or system change. The culture really doesn't change [31].

For all these reasons, it is not surprising that progress has been slow. From an historical perspective, however, a great deal has happened in a relatively short time. The vice grip of the dishonest and futile legal approach of deny and defend has been broken. Open communication and support are now at least part of the conversation in health-care organizations as the key organizations overseeing their behavior, AHRQ, NQF, TJC, CMS, ABMS, and ACGME, have incorporated it into their standards. The pace has accelerated. A better future is in sight for our patients and their doctors.

References

1. Iedema R, Allen S, Britton K, et al. Patients' and family members' views on how clinicians enact and how they should enact incident disclosure: the "100 patient stories" qualitative study. BMJ. 2011;343:d4423.
2. Vincent C, Young M, Phillips A. Why do people sue doctors? A study of patients and relatives taking legal action. Lancet. 1994;343:1609–14.
3. Gallagher TH, Waterman AD, Ebers AG, Fraser VJ, Levinson W. Patients' and physicians' attitudes regarding the disclosure of medical errors. JAMA. 2003;289:1001–7.
4. Hilfiker D. Facing our mistakes. N Engl J Med. 1984;310:118–22.
5. Vincent C. Research into medical accidents: a case of negligence? Br Med J. 1989;299:1150–3.
6. Wu A, Folkman S, McPhee S, et al. Do house officers learn from their mistakes? JAMA. 1991;265:2089–94.
7. Christensen J, Levinson W, Dunn P. The heart of darkness: the impact of perceived mistakes on physicians. J Gen Intern Med. 1992;7:424–31.
8. Studdert DM, Michelle MM, Gawande AA, Brennan TA, Wang YC. Disclosure of medical injury to patients: an improbable risk management strategy. Health Aff. 2007;26:215–26.
9. Kraman SS, Hamm G. Risk management: extreme honesty may be the best policy. Ann Intern Med. 1999;131:963–7.
10. Gallagher TH, Studdert D, Levinson W. Disclosing harmful medical errors to patients. N Engl J Med. 2007;356:2713–9.
11. Mello MM, Boothman RC, McDonald T, Driver J, Lembitz A, Bouwmeester D, Dunlap B, Gallagher T. Communication-and-resolution programs: the challenges and lessons learned from six early adopters. Health Aff (Millwood). 2014;33(1):20–9.

12. Kachalia A, Kaufman SR, Boothman R, et al. Liability claims and costs before and after implementation of a medical error disclosure program. Ann Intern Med. 2010;153:213–21.

13. Boothman CR, Imhoff JS, Campbell AD. Nurturing a culture of patient safety and achieving lower malpractice risk through disclosure: lessons learned and future directions. Front Health Serv Manag. 2012;28:13–28.

14. Gallagher TH, Levinson W. Disclosing harmful medical errors to patients: a time for professional action. Arch Intern Med. 2005;165:1819–24.

15. Clinton H, Obama B. Making patient safety the centerpiece of medical liability reform. N Engl J Med. 2006;354:2205–8.

16. MITSS: supporting patients and families for more than a decade. Patient Saf Qual Healthc. 2013. Accessed 4 June 2020, at https://www.psqh.com/analysis/mitss-supporting-patients-and-families-for-more-than-a-decade/.

17. When Things Go Wrong: Responding to Adverse Events. A consensus statement of the Harvard Hospitals. Massachusetts Coalition for the Prevention of Medical Errors: Boston; 2006.

18. National Quality Forum. Safe practices for better healthcare: 2006 update. Washington, DC: NQF; 2007.

19. The Joint Commission. Accreditation guide for hospitals. Oakbrook Terrace: The Joint Commission; 2011.

20. McDonald T, Helmchen L, Smith K, et al. Responding to patient safety incidents: the "seven pillars". Quality and Safety in Health Care. 2010;19:e11–e4.

21. Lambert BL, Centomani NM, Smith KM, et al. The "seven pillars" response to patient safety incidents: effects on medical liability processes and outcomes. Health Serv Res. 2016;51:2491–515.

22. Pillen M, Hayes E, Driver N, et al. Longitudinal evaluation of the patient safety and medical liability reform demonstration program: demonstration grants final evaluation report. Rockville: Agency for Healthcare Research and Quality; 2016. Report No.: AHRQ Publication No. 16-0038-2-EF.

23. Bell SK, Smulowitz PB, Woodward AC, et al. Disclosure, apology, and offer programs: stakeholders' views of barriers to and strategies for broad implementation. Milbank Q. 2012;90:682–705.

24. Acts of 2012, Chapter 224: an act improving the quality of health care and reducing costs through increased transparency, efficiency, and innovation. Section 221–223. Boston; The General Court of the Commonwealth of Massachusetts; 2012.

25. Kachalia A, Sands K, Van Niel M, et al. Effects of a communication-and-resolution program on hospitals' malpractice claims and costs. Health Aff. 2018;37:1836–44.

26. Mello MM, Kachalia A, Roche S, et al. Outcomes in two Massachusetts hospital systems give reason for optimism about communication-and-resolution programs. Health Aff. 2017;36:1795–803.

27. McDonald T, Niel M, Gocke H, Tarnow D, Hatlie M, Gallagher T. Implementing communication and resolution programs: lessons learned from the first 200 hospitals. J Patient Saf Risk Manag. 2018;23:73–8.

28. Boothman RC, Blackwell AC, Campbell DA Jr, Commiskey E, Anderson S. A better approach to medical malpractice claims? The University of Michigan experience. J Health Life Sci Law. 2009;2:125–59.

29. Boothman RC. CANDOR: the antidote to deny and defend? Health Serv Res. 2016;51:2487–90.

30. Communication and Optimal Resolution (CANDOR) Toolkit: Patient Safety Tools and Training Materials. Agency for Healthcare Research and Quality. Accessed 8 July 2020, at https://www.ahrq.gov/patient-safety/capacity/candor/modules.html.

31. Gallagher TH, Boothman RC, Schweitzer L, Benjamin EM. Making communication and resolution programmes mission critical in healthcare organisations. BMJ Qual Saf. 2020;29(11):875–8.

20

Ensuring Medical Competence of Physicians

Gwyneth Vives, a scientist at Los Alamos National Laboratory in New Mexico, suffered a complication and bled to death 3 hours after giving birth to a healthy boy in 2001. It was 4 days before Christmas. Vives suffered a vaginal tear and other lacerations during the delivery that caused profuse bleeding. Her obstetrician, Pamela Johnson, was sued for failure to order a blood transfusion for Vives as well as abandonment since she had turned over repair of the vaginal tear to a midwife. Two other patients also sued Johnson. Jean Challacombe alleged that Johnson tore her bowel and uterus while doing a dilation and curettage the same day Vives died. Tanya Lewis accused Johnson of doing an unnecessary hysterectomy.

Johnson had been forced to leave a previous job at Duke University Medical Center in North Carolina because of a "high surgical complication rate" and the "worst QA (quality assurance) file of anyone at Duke." At least three patients had filed claims against Johnson for malpractice. Later, Johnson lied to get her New Mexico license, saying she had never lost hospital privileges, according to an order of the New Mexico Medical Board [1].

"It's not bad people, it's bad systems," we said. But it has been a hard sell. When something bad happens, the natural reaction is to blame, to point the finger at the person who made the mistake, the bad doctor. We now know that this is both wrong and ineffective. Most harm, most errors—probably 95% or more—do, in fact, result from bad systems that lead good people to do bad things. That concept has been the main driver of patient safety: to get people to think of errors and harm as the result of faulty systems, not faulty people.

But there are some "faulty" people—doctors whose incompetence or negligence harms and kills patients. "That's not a systems problem," people would say. Ah, but it is. Our doctors are educated and trained by a system, certified by a system, monitored by a system, and disciplined by a system. What are those systems? And do they identify doctors when they begin to fail, assess them, and do something about it—*before* they hurt someone? A prevention system, or at least an early warning system. A reasonable question. Indeed, a vital question.

The System We Have

The system we have for producing a competent physician is composed of several interdependent systems. We have a rigorous *educational* system for medicine. Everyone knows that medical education is very difficult, intense, detailed, and challenging. Medical school is hard to get into, the bar is high, and graduates are well-equipped with scientific knowledge when they emerge. This is followed by 3–5 years of residency training and additional years of subspecialty fellowship training, essentially an in-hospital graded experience organized by specialty and culminating in examination and certification of competence by the specialty board ("Board certification").

The system for ensuring the *continuing* competence of the practicing physician also has several parts. The main responsibility falls to the individual specialty boards, who, in conjunction with their association, the American Board of Medical Specialties (ABMS), attempt to ensure continuing competence for the 85% of physicians who are certified by repeated assessments of their diplomates (the word for those certified) through maintenance of certification programs.

State licensing boards exercise responsibility for continuing competence of physicians through periodic relicensing. All but two rely largely on physicians certifying that they have completed a required number of continuing education courses and truthfully answering relicensing application questions about such things as malpractice claims, other civil lawsuits, criminal charges, illness and substance use, and even whether they have paid their taxes.

At the hospital or practice plan level, the system for ensuring continuing competence is *credentialing*, a process that determines whether a physician has admitting privileges to the hospital (or practice in a group) for their patients. Privileges are conferred annually or biannually by a committee of physician peers based on the recommendation of the department chair.

What's the Problem?

The problem is that these systems are not coordinated, and they don't work very well. Despite the many layers of responsibility and the array of mechanisms for ensuring safe and competent care, too many physicians fall short, and too many patients are harmed. Let's look at the facts.

Direct measures of physician performance are hard to come by. There is no nationally standardized system for routine measurement of outcomes of physicians' treatments. An indirect measure of incompetence is malpractice claims, but only claims that result in a payment to the patient are recorded, about a fifth of claims [2]. In 2019, 8378 payments were made for claims against physicians, down significantly from 16,116 in 2001 [3]. (Perhaps as the result of improved disclosure policies?—see Chap. 19.)

Another indirect measure is disciplinary actions by state medical boards. In 2017, 4081 physicians were disciplined by state medical board, including 1147 reprimanded (i.e., censured), 1343 restricted, and 264 who had their licenses revoked [4].

Malpractice claims and disciplinary actions by state boards capture only the proverbial tip of the iceberg. Most negligence is not reported, and few patients sue (see Chap. 1). For each of these cases, there are dozens that are not reported and many more instances of substandard care that results in patient harm.

More information is available about behavioral problems. Studies of disruptive behavior are disturbing. These include angry outbursts, verbal threats, shouting, swearing, degrading and demeaning comments, and threats of physical force, as well as shaming and sexual harassment [5].

Surveys of nurses show that more than 90% report experiencing such abuse [6], many of them repeatedly. Abuse of medical students is also common. Annual surveys of graduating medical students by the Association of American Medical Colleges (AAMC) show that 12–20% report abuse [7], although other data suggest it is much more common [8, 9]. In one survey of students from twenty-four different medical schools, 64% reported at least one incident of mistreatment by faculty, 76% by residents [10].

Residents in training are also victims. Half of 1791 residents in 1 survey reported being subjected to bullying, belittling, and humiliation [11]. A meta-analysis of 52 studies of residents showed that the prevalence of intimidation, harassment and discrimination was 64% [12].

Patients are also targets of abuse. Surveys show that 13–27% of patients report problems with doctor communication [13]. Patient interviews show the percentage is closer to 50% [14].

Why Doctors Fail

Why? Why do physicians who have successfully completed medical school and a rigorous residency training fail to maintain their competence or develop patterns of disruptive and unsafe behavior that compromise their ability to give high-quality, competent care? There are many reasons. Some succumb to the urge to establish a large practice to fulfill monetary needs or underlying feelings of inadequacy and then find its demands more than they can cope with. Others become overconfident and become unable to acknowledge shortcomings. Some are lazy and just don't keep up.

But for most, the causes are more mundane. Like everyone else, physicians have mental and physical health issues. Major depressive disorders occur in 16% of the public. The extent among physicians is unknown, but higher suicide rates—40% higher than the public for male physicians and 100% higher for female physicians—suggest depression is also probably more common [15].

The extent of physical illness among physicians is also unknown, but a reasonable estimate is that at least 10% of doctors must restrict their practices for several months or more at some time in their 40-year careers because of disabling illness [15]. Nor are physicians exempt from cognitive decline as they age, although we have no data.

Approximately 10–12% of physicians will develop a substance abuse problem at some time in their careers. About half of these are alcohol dependence, the rest, opioids and other drugs [16].

Stress is another factor. Physicians are subjected to unique stresses that can lead to dysfunctional behavior. Overwork, sleep deprivation, decreasing reimbursement, and pressure to see more patients are common. In recent years, the fraction of physicians exhibiting burnout has skyrocketed [17]. Young physicians worry about achieving a work/family balance and paying off their educational debts, which in 2018 averaged $196,520 at graduation. Stress leads to isolation and maladaptive coping strategies, such as alcohol or drug abuse.

Putting this all together, the conclusion is stunning. As John Fromson and I wrote in *Problem Doctors: Is There a Systems-Level Solution?*: "When all conditions are considered, **at least one third of all physicians will experience, at some time in their career, a period during which they have a condition that impairs their ability to practice medicine safely**" [15].

The question is: What do we do about it?

Who Is Responsible for Ensuring Physician Competence and Safety?

Who is responsible for making sure that physicians are competent and safe? The answer is disarmingly simple: physicians. Society has given physicians an implicit contract: it grants them incredible powers to cross otherwise sacrosanct boundaries—to learn our most intimate thoughts and invade our bodies and our psyches—in return for the pledge that the profession will use its knowledge and skills for the good of society. It grants the profession substantial autonomy to determine its own educational standards and the right of self-regulation.

The essence of medicine's contract with society is *professionalism*, the commitment of the physician to place the interests of the patient above their own, to maintain their skills, and to ensure that their colleagues do so as well [18].

One way physicians have met this obligation is through specialty societies, the AMA, and state medical societies, which from their origins have considered improving the quality of practice of their members their first priority—their purpose, really. The American College of Surgeons (ACS), for example, was the first to set standards for hospitals, leading ultimately to the formation of the Joint Commission.

Specialty society annual meetings are largely devoted to learning, both from formal instruction and from research presentations. Larger societies, such as the American College of Physicians, American Association of Family Practitioners, and American Society of Anesthesiologists, have extensive extramural continuing education programs and online resources. State medical societies also sponsor educational programs. These programs assist physicians in accruing specific hours of medical education that are required for relicensure by their state boards of medicine.

Physicians have also met their obligation by developing professional organizations that set standards and exercise oversight. The primary responsibility for ensuring physician competence in the USA rests with two national organizations: the American Board of Medical Specialties (ABMS), whose specialty boards examine and certify practicing physicians, and the Accreditation Council for Graduate Medical Education (ACGME), which sets standards and oversees physician residency education.

American Board of Medical Specialties

Specialty board certification is the essential badge of quality for physicians. For decades, becoming certified required only that the physician pass a rigorous written and oral examination at the conclusion of residency. You were certified for life. That began to change in 1969 when the newly formed Board of Family Medicine required that diplomates be reexamined every 10 years to maintain certified status. The process of recertification gradually spread to other specialties.

By the late 1990s, just as the patient safety movement was beginning to gain momentum, the leadership of the ABMS realized they needed to do much more to ensure their diplomates were competent and to assure the public that was so.

In a rather remarkable joint effort, ABMS and ACGME came together in 1999 to explicitly define physician competence. They described six domains of clinical competency that physicians would be expected to achieve and maintain [19] (Box 20.1). The six competencies were adopted by the individual specialty boards as the basis for assessments of physicians. The ACGME adopted them as the framework for progressive training in a specialty.

Box 20.1 Six Domains of Competency
- *Practice-based learning and improvement*: show an ability to investigate and evaluate patient care practices, appraise and assimilate scientific evidence, and improve the practice of medicine.
- *Patient care and procedural skills*: provide care that is compassionate, appropriate, and effective treatment for health problems and to promote health.
- *Systems-based practice*: demonstrate awareness of and responsibility to the larger context and systems of health care. Be able to call on system resources to provide optimal care (e.g., coordinating care across sites or serving as the primary case manager when care involves multiple specialties, professions. or sites).
- *Medical knowledge*: demonstrate knowledge about established and evolving biomedical, clinical, and cognate sciences and their application in patient care.
- *Interpersonal and communication skills*: demonstrate skills that result in effective information exchange and teaming with patients, their families, and professional associates (e.g., fostering a therapeutic relationship that is ethically sound, using effective listening skills with nonverbal and verbal communication, working as both a team member and at times as a leader).
- *Professionalism*: demonstrate a commitment to carrying out professional responsibilities, adherence to ethical principles, and sensitivity to diverse patient populations.

Adapted from Ref. [19]

In addition, the periodic recertification examinations would be replaced by continuing maintenance of certification (MOC), which required the physician to demonstrate a commitment to lifelong learning, self-evaluation, and improving their practice and to prove it through periodic assessments.

Each specialty board devised its own MOC program, tailoring the six competencies to its individual needs and defining how to meet the requirements. The certifying board would then "continually" determine whether or not the physician is in compliance with its MOC requirements. Finally, there was an answer to the patient's concern, "I know he was competent when he was certified, but is he competent now?"

Boards differed greatly in how they assessed compliance. For most, physicians were required to periodically document that they had maintained the core six competencies. A four-part assessment was designed to test their medical knowledge, clinical competence, communication skills, and quality of care. Approaches have included patient registries, audits, peer review, and comparison to national benchmarks. Another is to give credit for participating in hospital quality improvement projects.

Physicians pushed back. Naturally skeptical, they had to be convinced that the process was relevant to their practices and would improve quality of care at a time when they felt overworked and underpaid. However, by 2012 about half of all certified specialists had complied [20].

Older physicians who had been exempted from the 10-year relicensing requirement when it began also sat this one out. As of 2012, of the 66,689 diplomates of the American Board of Internal Medicine who held only the old time-unlimited certificates, only 1% chose to become recertified through MOC [20].

The concept of the six competencies was truly brilliant. Its explicit definitions made it possible to measure competence for the first time. The ACGME incorporated them in standards for residency training. Medical schools adopted them to structure curricula, and the Joint Commission made them requirements for hospital evaluation of their physicians. CMS gave physicians a bonus on their Medicare reimbursement if they participated in its Physician Quality Reporting System and MOC.

Accreditation Council for Graduate Medical Education

The other professional organization responsible for ensuring competence of physicians is the Accreditation Council for Graduate Medical Education (ACGME) . Not unlike the Joint Commission, the ACGME accreditation process had for years focused on structural aspects of training programs, such as qualifications of the program director and number of teaching cases, plus a few outcomes, especially the percentage of graduates who passed certifying examinations.

Following the development of the six competencies, ACGME in 2001 launched the Outcome Project, which requires residency training programs to configure curricula and evaluation processes in the framework of the six competencies.

In 2011, in conjunction with changes in duty hour limits, a major emphasis was begun to improve supervision and providing a safe and effective environment for care and learning: the Clinical Learning Environment Review (CLER) Program.

Through frequent site visits independent of the accreditation process, CLER focuses on the resident experience and progress in six areas: patient safety; health-care quality and reduction in health-care disparities; care transitions; supervision; fatigue management, mitigation, and duty hours; and professionalism [21]. "Milestones" were developed that describe the skills, knowledge, and behaviors in the six areas that residents are expected to reach at each level as they progress through their training.

These ACGME programs are described in greater detail in Chap. 18.

The Joint Commission

The Joint Commission plays an important role in enabling and ensuring physician competence through its oversight role with hospitals. Not only does it require hospitals to have systems and programs that foster quality and safety, which of necessity involve physicians, hospitals are also required to have programs to oversee and enhance physician performance. See Chap. 12 for more details.

State Licensing Boards

An interesting aspect of self-regulation is state regulation. While that sounds like an oxymoron, it is not. State medical licensing boards have legal authority to hold physicians accountable for competent practice, but for many years they were composed entirely of physicians, who were deemed the only ones qualified to judge other doctors. In recent years lay members have been added in some states, but physicians still dominate.

State boards exercise their authority primarily through licensing. Initial licensing for American medical school graduates requires passing three examinations taken in medical school and the first year of residency. Subsequently, physicians are required to complete a certain number of hours of continuing education annually and pay a fee to renew their licenses. State boards can also require physicians to undergo evaluations to ascertain knowledge and skill and require educational remediation and/or rehabilitation of physicians who have physical, mental, or substance use disorders.

Oversight is typically passive. Rather than actively monitoring or auditing performance of doctors in practice, boards tend to function in a reactive mode, responding to malpractice suits, patient complaints, and the occasional problem physician referred by a health-care organization.

State boards can place physicians on probation, censure, ask them to sign a letter of agreement to change behavior, restrict practice, or remove their license to practice. But they are reluctant to do so. Physicians on boards are very sympathetic to their colleagues, in part because they are aware of their own vulnerability. Of the nearly 600,000 physicians in practice in 2017, only 4081 (0.7%) were disciplined by their state boards [4].

Boards are particularly reluctant to take away licenses because doing so is an existential threat to the physician, rendering them unable to practice. As a result, it rarely happens. Licenses were suspended or revoked for 904 physicians (0.15%) in 2017 [4].

Boards also have a long history of being very forgiving of those with psychoactive substance use disorders. (William Halsted, legendary surgeon at Johns Hopkins Hospital and founder of the residency system, was a known cocaine addict.) Physicians with a substance use problem that interferes with their ability to practice medicine are usually required to enter into a 3–5-year monitoring agreement that includes mandatory random urine testing, workplace monitoring by peers and supervisors, attendance at meetings like A.A. or N.A., and seeing a therapist or alcohol/drug counselor. If they fail to follow through, they may have their license to practice suspended until a significant period of being clean and sober is once again documented.

While these practices accord with current thinking that addiction is a disease and not a moral failing, the difference from other fields, of course, is that impaired physicians put patients at risk. Forgiveness can be carried to extremes. For example, a Virginia psychiatrist was in drug rehabilitation 9 times and relapsed at least 12 times during a 10-year period before the medical board took away her license [22]. In a five-year period, only 1400 physicians across the country were disciplined for substance abuse and reported to the National Practitioner Data Bank [23].

The National Practitioner Data Bank was established by Congress in 1986 to stop doctors from escaping troubled histories by having a central location where any sanctions or malpractice verdicts could be recorded. Names are not made public, but they are available to state licensing boards, hospitals, and other health-care entities, including federal agencies, who are required to consult NPDB prior to hiring.

Nevertheless, hospitals and boards have dragged their feet on complying, reluctant to tarnish a physician's reputation or restrict their ability to practice. Various tactics are employed to circumvent the requirement to report physicians, most commonly the hospital rather than the physician paying the settlement in a malpractice case.

Nearly 54 percent of all hospitals have never reported a disciplinary action to the data bank. For example, in the Vives case mentioned above, no one told the data bank that Pamela Johnson had been forced to leave her job at Duke. Enforcement is no better: no fine or penalty has ever been levied according to the federal Department of Health and Human Services, which oversees the system.

Federation of State Medical Boards

The national voice for state boards is the Federation of State Medical Boards (FSMB). All 71 state medical and osteopathic boards are members. The FSMB is the spokesperson for issues related to regulation and discipline. It proposes policy changes and facilitates collaborative efforts of state boards and other entities. With the National Board of Medical Examiners (NBME), it sponsors the US Medical Licensing Examination that is required of all medical school graduates for medical licensure.

FSMB recommends standards, but it has no enforcement power. In 2004, it promoted a radically new policy—"State medical boards have a responsibility to the public to ensure the ongoing competence of physicians seeking re-licensure"—i.e., meaningful maintenance of licensure like the maintenance of certification programs that were being developed [24].

In 2010, FSMB expanded this to declare that as a condition of license renewal, physicians provide evidence of participation in a program of professional development and lifelong learning based on the six ABMS competencies [25].

It then took the step that quality and safety experts had long called for to align licensing and certification: participation in the MOC process of their specialty board would satisfy the standards for relicensure [26].

FSMB also plays a key role in the assessment and rehabilitation of problem doctors. While many state medical societies have monitoring programs for doctors with alcohol and substance use disorders, fewer address knowledge and skill deficits, personality disorders, technical and cognitive deficiencies, or disruptive behavior.

A joint program of FSMB and NBME, the *Post-Licensure Assessment System* (PLAS), administers a standardized examination of clinical knowledge to physicians referred by state medical boards or by themselves. If results are unsatisfactory, the physician may undergo an additional assessment and then choose (or be required) to participate in a remediation program [27].

Alternatively, physicians may be evaluated by the Physician Assessment and Clinical Education (PACE) Program, founded in 1966 at UC San Diego School of Medicine long before FSMB took on this responsibility. The program assesses physicians referred by state boards as a condition of maintaining their licenses. It conducts a rigorous evaluation of a physician's ability to safely practice medicine. They undergo an oral clinical examination, clinical observation, and physical and mental health screening. PACE offers remedial courses in anger management, communication, professional boundaries, prescribing, and medical record keeping [28].

A number of other programs have been developed in recent years for doctors and other professionals with problems. For all, the goal is to enable dyscompetent professionals to undergo remediation and training so that they can remain in practice.

Unfortunately, there are many barriers to physicians' participation in these programs. Foremost are financial. In our fee-for-service health-care system, the physician is in a triple bind. Not only do they lose income while undergoing rehabilitation, they often have to pay a substantial fee for it, and if they are absent for more than a few weeks, their practice deteriorates as patients find other doctors. In a more rational system, their employer would maintain their salary and pay the costs of rehabilitation.

Another problem is that if residency retraining is needed, it is difficult to find programs that are willing and able to add the physician to their roster of residents, even for a short time. Similarly, their colleagues and hospital may be reluctant to take on responsibility or potential liability for supervising their practice. Doctors are uncomfortable supervising their peers.

Experience shows that performance problems can be solved or significantly ameliorated for the vast majority of physicians. Few need to be, nor should be, removed from practice. We know what to do.

Making it happen is another matter. Rehabilitation and remediation are still very much a work in progress.

New York Cardiac Advisory Committee

Perhaps the most effective—and unique—instrument of state regulation is the New York Cardiac Advisory Committee. In the 1950s, long before there was national interest in improving quality or safety, the Health Department of New York convened a group of respected cardiac surgeons and cardiologists to oversee the newly developing field of cardiac surgery. The committee was an outgrowth of the state certificate of need program that regulated which hospitals could establish new programs. It had the power to limit the number of hospitals performing cardiac surgery. Its responsibility was to establish and maintain high-quality programs geographically distributed to meet the needs of the state's population.

In 1989, responding to the concern that its comparisons of mortality among hospitals were not valid because they were not adjusted for risk, and recognizing the need for a data-based approach, the CAC established the Cardiac Surgical Reporting System (CSRS) to develop risk-adjusted measures and collect data on outcomes of coronary artery bypass graft (CABG) surgery. For the first time, the adjusted outcomes of all cardiac surgeons and all hospitals performing cardiac surgery were measured and reported publicly.

The initial findings showed wide variations in 30-day operative mortality with low-volume surgeons and low-volume hospitals faring the worst. High-outlier hospitals were put on probation. The responses were prompt. The survival of their programs at risk, most of them undertook a variety of actions to improve their programs: establishing full-time chiefs, replacing chiefs and poor-performing surgeons, adding cardiac anesthesiologists and nurse specialists, etc. The results were dramatic. Within 3 years, mortality dropped 41%, giving New York the lowest CABG mortality of any state, a status it has maintained [29].

The reports attracted intense media attention in the early years, causing concern about shaming and government interference. Mortality for hospitals and surgeons were reported in the newspapers.

Was that appropriate? Certainly, the public has a right to know. This notion, now well-accepted and enshrined in Hospital Compare and other public data, was a radical idea at the time and hotly debated. There is little question, however, that the public release of the information was a key motivator for change.

As the CAC began to measure risk-adjusted outcomes of CABG surgery in 1989, they approached our team at RAND to do an appropriateness study of CABG, angioplasty, and coronary angiography. Our earlier work had shown high rates of inappropriate use of these procedures. The CAC and the state health department wanted to know if their efforts resulted in lower rates in New York. With their collaboration we were able to get funding for the study, which we carried out over the next 2 years.

The results confirmed the higher quality of cardiac surgical care in New York. The inappropriate rate for CABG was 2.4%, far lower than the 14% found in a previous study in several other states. Mortality was also low, 2.0%, far lower than the national average of 5.5%. The inappropriate use rate for angioplasty was also low: 4%. These added to the evidence that close oversight and the feedback of risk-adjusted data are powerful motivators for quality [30–32].

The CAC program has continued to be successful. It is a superb example of the power of intelligent, well-managed regulation to ensure quality and safety of health care. Unlike other states, in New York the health commissioner has the authority to require reporting, to carry out audits to verify data quality, and to establish the oversight committee and the power to shut programs down.

Involving the state's leading cardiac surgeons and cardiologists in the advisory committee gave credibility to its decisions and acceptability to the cardiac surgical community. The focus on objective evidence provided a powerful incentive for poor performers to improve [29]. The program is a model of effective regulation.

The Civil Justice System—Malpractice Litigation

Finally, when all else fails, the legal system steps in. Doctors can be sued and forced to pay substantial compensation if their performance can be proven to be negligent. The legal definition of negligence is quite simple: failure to meet the standard of care. Proving that is another matter. In the end, relatively few patients are compensated. The Harvard Medical Practice Study found that fewer than 10% of patients harmed by negligent care ever sued [33]. National studies show that fewer than half of malpractice suits result in a payment to the patient [2, 34].

But negligent care is only responsible for a small fraction of serious medical injury. The vast majority of injured patients have no recourse to the legal system. Malpractice litigation also fails to achieve its other purported objective: deterring bad behavior in the future. There is no evidence this happens. Physicians see cases as one off, bad luck, and unjustified. They often don't believe they have done anything wrong. The process of being sued is devastating for physicians, however, as is discussed in more detail in Chap. 19.

A serious defect of the current system is that malpractice settlements are usually sealed, prohibiting any party from making the information accessible. Not only does this cloak of secrecy prevent the medical team from learning from the event and fixing the faulty systems, it keeps vital information away from state boards and future patients.

Overall, malpractice litigation is an ineffective tool for ensuring or improving physician competence. Interestingly, fewer patients are suing. Malpractice payments dropped from 16,116 in 2001 to 8378 in 2019 [3]. It is tempting to attribute this to a reduction in patient injuries or to improved disclosure practices, but there is little evidence for either.

A far better legal approach would be *enterprise liability*, in which the institution, not the physician, is responsible for compensating patients for the costs of harm. Hospitals and health-care organizations would be sued instead. It makes sense. If, as we maintain, harm results from failed systems (including systems for ensuring physician competence), then it is the party responsible for the systems—the organization—that should be held accountable for their failures. Indeed, if we were really serious about this, we would require hospitals to compensate patients for *all* costs of the harm we have caused, even when no error is identified: no-fault compensation—as was recommended by the Harvard Medical Practice Study 30 years ago.

Hospital Responsibility for Physician Performance

As in politics, all quality is local. Medical specialty boards set standards, examine, and certify; states license and discipline; but meaningful oversight of physician performance, what happens in everyday practice, takes place where care is delivered. For 80% of physicians, that is the hospital. For others it can be their large multispecialty group. But for practitioners in solo or small group practice, such as primary care, psychiatry, and dermatology, oversight is often quite lax.

Hospital oversight is through *credentialing* committees, groups of physicians appointed by the medical staff who annually or biannually decide on admitting privileges and what procedures a doctor may perform. It is awesome power, second only to state licensing. If they are unable to admit patients to a hospital, most physicians cannot practice. They are professionally dead. Every hospital has a credentialing committee. Medical specialty boards are the carrot, credentialing committees are the stick.

The process that most credentialing committees use for carrying out this responsibility is quite simple: they rely on the recommendation from the specialty department chair. Typically, this is a pro forma process unless the department chair recommends against it. Then it can get very messy.

So, where "the rubber hits the road," where the action takes place to ensure physician competence, is the department. The department chair is ultimately responsible for assessing the competence of every member of the department. How do they do it?

Until very recently, assessment has been informal, especially in smaller private hospitals where the chair has little authority. The chair relied on personal knowledge about the physician and feedback from peers. Absent serious complaints from patients or staff about the physician's conduct, approval was routine.

Few department chairs actually reviewed patient outcomes or conducted peer assessment of performance. Annual physical examinations are still not required. Random drug testing is rare and hotly resisted by many physicians as an affront to their professionalism. Cognitive testing is almost nonexistent.

The good news is that methods for monitoring clinical performance have improved greatly in recent years. To be objective, evaluation must be based on data: compliance with standard practices and outcomes, how well patients do. While measuring outcomes is easiest with surgical patients, many "medical" outcomes are now also collected routinely. Individual results can then be compared with national and local norms to identify outliers who need attention.

The Joint Commission now requires that physicians currently on staff have an annual Ongoing Professional Practice Evaluation (OPPE). This is a summary of ongoing data collected for the purpose of assessing a practitioner's clinical competence and professional behavior. Newly hired physicians and those already on staff found to have competency issues on their OPPE are required to have a Focused Professional Practice Evaluation in which the medical staff evaluates the privilege-specific competence of the practitioner [35].

Psychosocial aspects of physician competence—communication skills, interpersonal relations, and ability to collaborate—have long been considered unquantifiable. They have traditionally been assessed informally through conversations with peers and coworkers. Personality or interest tests and the like have been tried and found not to be reliable. But one method of evaluation does produce data that is reliable and has proven to be quite useful: multisource feedback, popularly called "360" evaluations.

Multisource Feedback

Multisource feedback (MSF) is a formalized method of obtaining feedback about an individual's performance from those with whom they interact. Since the late 1990s, it has been used to assess physicians by Lockyer in the Physician Achievement Review (PAR) program in Alberta, Canada [36], but is now being increasingly used in US hospitals. The PACE program in California has used it for some time to evaluate physicians referred for problem behavior.

The process begins by having the physician and their peers, nurses, residents, and patients complete a questionnaire of 10–40 items that assess clinical behaviors, such as communication, collaboration, professionalism, interpersonal, and management skills. Typically, 7–15 individuals in each of these groups complete the questionnaire, rating the physician on a five-point scale. The results are tabulated by group, and mean scores are compared to the physician's self-assessment for each item. The department chairman then reviews the data with the physician to identify areas for improvement. Studies have shown that MSF has high reliability, validity, and feasibility [37].

The impact of the 360 review can be very powerful. In a pilot study some years ago in one department in a Boston hospital, we found that, as in Lake Wobegon, all physicians rated themselves above average for almost all questions. Peers tended to agree, but resident and nurse ratings were sometimes quite a bit lower, especially regarding interpersonal relations. Feedback of this information to the physician was always a surprise and sometimes emotionally very disturbing. Several were reduced to tears. It was a powerful motivation for change.

MSF is increasingly being used in the USA. ABMS now recommends that specialty boards use MSF to assess professionalism and knowledge, and ACGME requires training programs to use multiple evaluators to provide objective performance evaluation of residents. The Pulse 360 Program creates and sells 360 feedback tools and training programs for health care. It is used in over 200 hospitals [38].

Support of Physicians with Problems

With the demands of MOC, methods for evaluation and support are improving. Specialty boards, especially the ABIM, have become more engaged with hospitals in providing continuing education, translating standards into practice, and collecting outcome data to measure performance. Blue Cross Blue Shield Association, CIGNA HealthCare, Humana, and Wellpoint have incorporated them in their quality recognition programs.

But serious behavioral problems are often managed poorly. Department chairs may lack the training and skills to deal with them. Many fear confrontation and avoid it if possible. Peers are reluctant to be involved, valuing their own independence and respecting that of others.

A major barrier is that disciplinary action will often be vigorously resisted by the offending physician, who may even sue the department or the hospital. This leads to bad publicity in the newspapers and requires a number of doctors to spend many hours in depositions or hearings—a messy business, indeed. No wonder doctors shy away from judging their peers.

How Should it Work? The Ideal System

There must be a better way to ensure physician competence and improve quality of care. There is. It is for the hospital (or practice) to perform a meaningful evaluation of every physician every year using a routine, formal, proactive system of monitoring with validated measures, followed by action to remedy shortcomings when they are discovered. Some years ago, John Fromson and I proposed that the system must have three characteristics [15]:

- First, it must be *objective*, i.e., assessment must be based on data: patient outcomes data and compliance with performance standards, not on subjective judgments of personality or motivation.
- Second, it must be *fair*. All physicians in the organization must be evaluated by the same system, not just suspect individuals.
- Third, it must be *responsive*. When problems are identified, they must be treated promptly. There is no point in evaluation if nothing comes of it. Most physicians with problems will only need feedback. They can and will self-correct. Others may need counseling. Some may require referral to an outside program for assessment. Retraining may be needed.

An effective system is proactive. It is based on the notion that subpar performance can be objectively defined, routine monitoring can detect problems early, and the responses to deficiencies will be prompt and constructive.

The point is not to identify "bad apples" and throw them out, but to detect deficiencies early and correct them before patients are harmed, to enable good doctors with minor problems to become better, and to help those with more serious problems to overcome them if possible.

In the ideal system, the department adopts explicit standards, requires compliance, monitors performance, and responds to deficiencies. The department chair reviews performance data with each physician annually, and together they work out a plan for improvement as needed. In some cases, this may require external testing and remediation.

A similar oversight process should be required of larger medical groups and employed physicians. The remaining small number of physicians in solo or small practice might then be required by licensing authorities to take advantage of some mechanism like PACE or CPEP in order to maintain licensure.

Fortunately, as we have seen, the ABMS and specialty boards have worked hard in recent years to develop national standards of competence and behavior and to integrate them into the process of continuing certification. Closer coordination of this oversight with local review and response would lead to greater accountability and improved performance.

Nonregulatory Approaches to Improving Competence

Independent of the impressive changes to improve accountability by the establishment organizations described above, a number of independent voluntary initiatives have taken place over the years to improve the process of physician assessment and improvement. Several deserve special mention.

National Surgical Quality Improvement Program

In 1986, responding to a series of newspaper articles about poor care in Veterans Health Administration (VHA) hospitals, Congress mandated that VHA report risk-adjusted surgical outcomes annually and compare them to national averages. There was a problem, though: there were no known national averages and no known risk adjustment models!

But the VA was uniquely suited to develop them for its population. The VHA is the largest health-care provider in the USA, serving several million veterans and performing surgery in 128 of its 159 Veterans Administration Medical Centers (VAMCs). At the behest of their surgical leadership, a research group at the Brockton/West Roxbury VA Medical Center in Massachusetts led by Shukri Khuri, Chief of Surgery, and Jennifer Daley, an experienced quality-of-care researcher, carried out the National VA Surgical Risk Study from 1991 to 1993. Using data collected from 117,000 major operations in 44 VAMCs, they developed risk adjustment models for 30-day mortality and morbidity rates for noncardiac surgery [39].

They then turned their attention to measurement of surgical outcomes. Surgery is uniquely suitable for measurement of outcomes since there is a clearly defined expected outcome for every operation. Using this validated model for risk adjustment, outcomes could now be measured with some confidence in their validity.

In 1994 the VHA established the National VA Surgical Quality Improvement Program (NSQIP), a reporting and managerial structure for the continuous monitoring and enhancement of the quality of surgical care, under an executive committee led by Khuri and Daley [40].

Surgical clinical nurse reviewers (SCNRs) were trained in the accurate collection and timely transmission of risk adjustment data, consisting of 45 presurgical variables, 17 surgical variables, and 33 outcomes. Logistic regression analysis was used to calculate a predicted probability of 30-day mortality and complications. Risk-adjusted observed versus expected (O/E) outcome ratios were calculated for all types of procedures at the surgical service of each VAMC and overall.

Feedback of these procedure-specific O/E ratios is provided annually to the chief of surgery, director, and chief of staff of each VAMC, and the CMO of each Veterans Integrated Service Networks (VISN), as well as results for all participating hospitals, by code. Hospital leaders know only the code for their hospital.

The executive committee produces an annual assessment of high and low outliers and communicates levels of concern about high outlier status to hospital and VISN, as well as praise and rewards to low outliers. Persistent high outliers are subject to internal and external reviews.

NSQIP also develops and disseminates self-assessment tools to providers and managers and, at the request of a VAMC, organizes consultative site visits to assess data quality and performance.

NSQIP provides management (directors and CMOs of VISN) with advice and expertise in conducting external reviews and site visits and disseminates best practices reported by low O/E hospitals.

The first assessment of results showed that during the period from 1991 to 1997 30-day mortality decreased from 3.1 to 2.8 and morbidity decreased from 17.4 to 10.3. By 2006, postoperative mortality had dropped by 47% and morbidity rates by 43% [41].

The program was well-accepted by the chiefs of surgery who valued the feedback and learned to find and improve deficiencies. From the beginning, NSQIP has been about quality improvement, not judgment. The emphasis is on systems not providers. No individual provider-specific data is transmitted to the central data base.

Several aspects of NSQIP accounted for its success. Most important was the fact that VHA had in place a universal computerized record system, VISTA, that made clinical and laboratory data available for risk analysis. It also had access to the operating room log in every VAMC, so all procedures were automatically and reliably identified.

Second, for data entry it relied exclusively on trained surgical clinical nurse reviewers (SCNRs) who were experienced in practice, data collection, and quality assurance. This gave high levels of credibility, reliability, and validity to the data. Third, inclusion of surgical leaders from the field in the design of the program and oversight led to support by VAMC senior surgeons, administrators, VISN directors, and CMOs.

The private sector took notice. Why not use NSQIP for non-VA surgical departments? Within months of the first report, in 1999, a pilot program was begun in three academic surgical centers, University of Michigan, Emory University, and the University of Kentucky, to determine if the risk adjustment models would work for the more heterogeneous private sector patient populations. They did. Comparison of findings in 2747 patients at these centers with contemporary results in 41,360 patients in the VHA showed no differences in risk-adjusted mortality between the non-VA and VA cohorts [42].

Following this success, the American College of Surgeons (ACS) in 2001 sponsored a pilot program funded by AHRQ in18 private sector hospitals that showed that NSQIP also led to reduced morbidity and mortality in private sector hospitals. In 2004, ACS began enrolling additional private sector hospitals into ACS NSQIP. Within a year, 41 hospitals had joined. By 2018, participants included 568 hospitals in the USA, 96 in Canada, and 38 overseas. Nine of the top 10 hospitals ranked as America's Best Hospitals by *U.S. News & World Report* in 2018 participated in ACS NSQIP [41].

Meanwhile, NSQIP continues to work on improving. More specialty variables were incorporated; additional outcome measurements, such as functional status, quality of life, and patient satisfaction, were developed and incorporated; and structure and process measures were added [43].

Analysis of Patient Complaints

In the early 1990s, Gerald Hickson, Associate Dean for Clinical Affairs at Vanderbilt University Medical Center, and his colleagues found that analysis of written complaints by patients to the hospital was a useful tool for identifying physicians with interpersonal problems. About 2/3 of complaints were about a hospital or practice service or system issue; 1/3 were about a named physician.

While patients often complain about their doctors, it is unusual for them to make a formal complaint in writing [44]; most physicians receive none or only one or two over their entire professional career. But some have more. Hickson wondered if there was a relationship between the number of complaints and the likelihood of the physician being sued. ("Claims" in risk management parlance.)

Indeed, there was. In a six-year period, he found no claims for 81% of doctors who had only one or no complaints. The majority of those with 2–6 complaints also had no claims. But physicians with 4 or more complaints over this period were 16 times more likely to have 2 or more claims than physicians with no complaints. Those with 25 claims or more had a 95% chance of being sued [45].

Hickson realized that patient reports could serve as the basis of an "early warning system" to more rapidly identify and engage with physicians before harm occurred and suits began to accumulate. They could then be helped to overcome their deficiencies. He developed a tiered intervention program, the Promoting Professionalism Pyramid, that defined a process that started with a conversation with a colleague and escalated if needed to formal evaluation and required behavioral change.

Following the first complaint, a colleague would have a "cup of coffee conversation" in which the complaint is shared with the physician in a nonjudgmental way and they are asked to reflect on the event. Often the physician has not recognized the bad behavior and justifies it because of the situation. The colleague makes no judgment, merely delivering the news. But for many, that is all that is necessary: their behavior changes.

At the second level, when there have been additional reports that suggest a pattern of inappropriate behavior, an *awareness* intervention is called for. A respected colleague presents the data to the individual showing how their complaint history compares to that of their peers and gives them the opportunity to respond. Again, in most cases this is all that is needed to lead the physician to change behavior.

For those that do not respond to the awareness intervention, the response moves to the next level. The department chair steps in and makes it clear that the individual must change their behavior. Chairs are trained to work with the physician to define an improvement plan that may range from coaching and counseling to formal outside evaluation and retraining.

If the physician is unwilling to undergo assessment and take responsibility for improving, or if these measures fail, then disciplinary action is required, which can include revoking admitting privileges or reporting to the state medical board [46]. Fewer than 1% fall into this category.

Hickson also developed a comprehensive program at Vanderbilt to reduce disruptive behavior by teaching interpersonal skills and professionalism at all levels: medical students, residents, and physicians. Physician leaders also receive skills training for conducting interventions [46].

He also developed a Comprehensive Assessment Program for Professionals to provide medical and psychological evaluation and treatment planning. Group classes were developed for disruptive behavior, prescribing problems and crossing sexual boundaries [47].

National Alliance for Physician Competence

This was one of the most unusual and exciting ventures I was ever part of, both for its goal, which was to set standards for good medical practice, and for those who participated, who were leaders of the national groups that could make it happen—in education, regulation, professional societies, and others. It was also one of the most frustrating.

The Alliance was organized by James Thompson, President and CEO of the FSMB, an ENT physician and former Dean at Wake Forest School of Medicine. Moved by the IOM reports, *To Err is Human* and *Crossing the Quality Chasm*, Thompson recognized when he took over FSMB that state medical licensing boards needed better methods for determining physician competence, both for licensing and for disciplinary actions. ACGME and ABMS had defined the six competencies, and the ABMS was moving to maintenance of certification. Shouldn't state boards do likewise?

Thompson encouraged the Federation to issue a statement on the need for maintenance of licensure, but much more was needed to make it a reality. He conferred with experts he knew as a former Dean: Donald Melnick, President and CEO of the National Board of Medical Examiners (NBME); James Hallock, CEO of the Educational Commission for Foreign Medical Graduates (ECFMG); and David Leach, CEO of ACGME. They supported his effort but felt that a comprehensive strategy linking licensure to education and specialty certification was needed. The time had come to begin a dialogue about the future of physician education and self-regulation.

On March 24, 2005, they brought together more than 60 leaders and representatives from organized medicine, academic medicine, hospitals, regulatory agencies, the insurance industry, accrediting organizations, payers, and the public in Fort Worth, Texas, for the first "Summit" on Physician Accountability for Physician Competence (PA4PC) (Table 20.1). The goals were to determine (1) how to define a competent physician, (2) how to measure competency, and (3) how medical organizations would assure the public that physicians are maintaining competence throughout the lifetime of their practice [26].

With help from Innovation Labs, and financial support from the NBME, the meeting explored the context within which physicians

Table 20.1 Institutional members of the National Alliance for Physician Competence

The Association of American Medical Colleges
AARP
Accreditation Council for Continuing Medical Education
Accreditation Council for Graduate Medical Education
American Board of Internal Medicine Foundation
American Board of Medical Specialties
American Medical Association
American Osteopathic Association
American Osteopathic Board of Emergency Medicine
Association of American Medical Colleges
Association for Hospital Medical Education
Blue Cross/Blue Shield Association
Christiana Care
Council of Medical Specialty Societies
Crozer-Keystone Health System
Educational Commission for Foreign Medical Graduates
The Federation of State Medical Boards
Iowa Board of Medical Examiners
Michigan Board of Medicine
National Board of Medical Examiners
National Board of Osteopathic Medical Examiners
Oregon Board of Medical Examiners
The Robert Wood Johnson Foundation
Texas A&M Health Science Center

would be expected to demonstrate accountability in the year 2020. What should the system look like? The group was energized and quickly found common ground on the big issues.

In subsequent meetings, other relevant stakeholders, such as patients and content experts like myself, were added to the group. Over the next 2 years, in a series of semi-annual meetings PA4PC drafted detailed definitions of competence and the content for a document, Good Medical Practice, that described the behaviors and values one should expect of a competent physician. A task force worked on simplifying physicians' access to credentialing information for multiple purposes such as licensing and board certification. The group renamed itself the National Alliance on Physician Competence.

The good practice document was our central focus. It was based on the work of the General Medical Council in the UK but reframed in terms of the six domains of competency defined by ABMS and ACGME. There were great debates about terminology. Should the document say doctors "should" do such and such or "must" do it? Ultimately, both were rejected. This would be a statement of who we *are* and what we do—who we *aspire* to be—not because it is required, but because of our values and commitment to our professionalism. We would use simple declarative sentences: "We respect each patient's dignity and individuality"; "We promptly modify our practice to incorporate evidence-based care"; "We apologize promptly to a patient when an error has occurred."

As it came into focus, we realized that the document should begin with The Patient's Perspective: a comprehensive statement of what patients have a right to expect from doctors regarding medical knowledge and skills, communication and interpersonal skills, shared decision-making, access and availability, and ethical integrity. This is the lens through which we see our role, our duty. The *purpose* of competence is to provide optimal patient care.

We finished the first draft, Version 0.1, of *Good Medical Practice – USA*, on August 15, 2007. It described the behaviors expected of all doctors who are permitted to practice medicine. The Patient's Perspective was followed by Duties of the Doctor consisting of one chapter for each of the six domains of competency. It was incredibly detailed, 200 statements in all, providing guidance on every aspect of practice, especially those that are difficult, such as knowing one's limits, giving bad news, dealing with problem colleagues, etc. Simple declarative statements of what good doctors do.

We called on medical educators and regulators to incorporate these principles in everything they do and challenged all physicians to take personal responsibility for making it happen.

The Alliance grappled with the relationship between maintenance of licensure and maintenance of certification and how to engage the practicing community and the public in the effort. To facilitate the licensing and certification processes, it developed a standardized, comprehensive "Trusted Agent/Portfolio System" that would enable physicians to retrieve all needed credentials from a single source.

The Alliance examined how a "continuum of competence" could be established: a system that would start in medical school and continue through residency programs, licensure, specialty certification, hospital credentialing and privileging, and the accreditation of institutions. How would the use of Good Medical Practice and the Trusted Agent/Portfolio System impact long-term maintenance of competency throughout a physician's career?

The last meeting of the National Alliance for Physician Competence Summit was held on July 7–9, 2008. The goal was to prepare to go public. Small groups synthesized and polished models to shift the paradigm for competence. These were then rolled into a single model of 14 components. Others focused on finalizing the renamed *Guide to Good Medical Practice*. Plans were made to "go live" with it in September, when Alliance participants would distribute the document. A draft Alliance website was created. A revised Alliance Participant Agreement was approved.

Then it all fell apart. From the beginning, the AMA had been a reluctant participant. It traditionally opposed anyone telling doctors how to practice and was against giving state boards more power. It declared opposition to the Guide even before it was

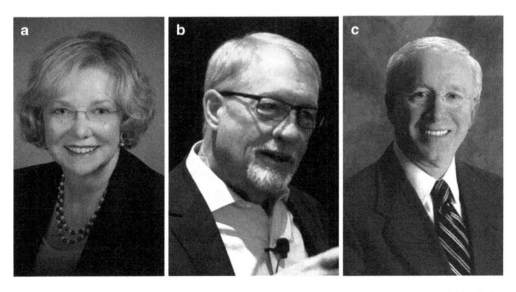

(**a**) Jennifer Daley, (**b**) Jerry Hickson, and (**c**) Jim Thompson. (All rights reserved)

written, maintaining that medicine is full of gray areas that are too difficult to measure. It opposed the concept of maintenance of certification.

At the last two meetings, it sought to undermine the process of the meetings by sending a large number of delegates who raised objections in all the working sessions. Although most of these were rejected by the majority, they disrupted the collaborative process.

Finally, at the last session the AMA withdrew its support. And, much to my surprise, despite the fact that it was the convener, so did the FSMB. It was proving to be too much for the individual state licensing boards. They were reluctant to take on this level of responsibility, and they saw no way to obtain the resources that would be required. The ABMS did not fight for it. It was having enough trouble figuring out how to implement the six competencies. The Alliance was finished. Our "brief shining moment," our Camelot, was over.

The Coalition for Physician Accountability

But Don Melnick, Jim Hallock, and Darrell Kirsch, CEO of the AAMC, were not going to let the concept die. The next year, they formed the Coalition for Physician Accountability to continue the discussion and further the cause. Its membership includes the stakeholders who have direct responsibility for assessment, accreditation, licensure, and certification along the continuum of medical education and practice.

The Coalition provides a forum for dialogue about ways to "promote professional accountability by improving the quality, efficiency, and continuity of the education, training and assessment of physicians" [48]. The Coalition meets twice yearly to analyze critical issues related to the regulation of physician education and practice and to develop consensus on actions to address them.

It functions through its member's endorsement of consensus statements about a diverse group of topics: regulation, innovation in medical school curricula, graduate medical education accreditation, interprofessional education, medical student and physician burnout, use of health information technology, opioid epidemic mitigation, interstate licensure, and a framework for professional competence and lifelong learning. It developed a consensus letter that was sent to Congress regarding maintaining Medicare support of GME, and it sent a letter to the National Coordinator outlining the commitment of Coalition members to promoting the use of health information technology.

Conclusion

Ensuring physician competence is a complex and difficult business. Despite the huge amount of work done by many diverse parties, it is still very much a work in progress. Oversight bodies, the state licensing boards and, especially, the specialty boards, have made substantial improvements in how they function, but the results still fall far short of achieving their objectives.

Why? Why doesn't the system work better? Why don't ABMS and the specialty boards make it work better and require, audit, and enforce adherence to the impressive and innovative processes they developed for maintenance of certification based on the six competencies?

Undoubtedly, there are many reasons, but I suggest that the fundamental reason, the "root cause" if you will, is that it is contrary to human nature for any group to police itself. We have not asked that of the other major industries where safety is critical: aviation and nuclear power. They are closely regulated by specific government agencies.

Do we need a federal agency to regulate quality and safety in health care? I have long believed we do [49]. The federal agencies regulating aviation and nuclear power are good models. The government exercises strict oversight of compliance with its rules, but those rules were developed in collaboration with the industry. Participation leads to buy-in and higher likelihood of compliance. (Recall the New York Cardiac Advisory Committee.) An agency developing regulations for doctors should collaborate with the specialty boards and state boards as well as representatives from professional societies and health-care organizations.

Hospitals should be held accountable for their physicians' performance. They should participate in developing regulations that ensure they are accountable to the public, such as required reporting of adverse events. The Joint Commission should be a partner in this process and play an important role by carrying out the necessary annual or semi-annual audits.

We have made tremendous progress in recent years in defining competence and measuring it. What was formerly implicit and casual can now be defined in an explicit and formal manner. We now know how to enable physicians to realize their full potential and by so doing immensely improve the quality and safety of patient care. The time has come to make it happen.

References

1. Thompson CW. Poor performance records are easily outdistanced. The Washington Post; April 12, 2005.
2. Studdert DM, Mello MM, Gawande AA, et al. Claims, errors, and compensation payments in medical malpractice litigation. N Engl J Med. 2006;354:2024–33.
3. National Practitioner Data Bank (2020): Adverse action and medical malpractice reports (1990 - March 31, 2020). U.S. Department of Health and Human Services, Health Resources and Services Administration, Bureau of Health Workforce, Division of Practitioner Data Bank; 2020.
4. Federation of State Medical Boards. U.S. Medical Regulatory Trends and Actions 2018. Euless, Texas: Federation of State Medical Boards; 2018.
5. Leape L, Shore M, Dienstag J, et al. A culture of respect: I. The nature and causes of disrespectful behavior. Acad Med. 2012;87:845–52.
6. Saxton R, Hines T, Enriquez M. The negative impact of nurse-physician disruptive on patient safety: a review of the literature. J Patient Saf. 2009;5:180–3.
7. Mavis B, Sousa A, Lipscomb W, Rappley MD. Learning about medical student mistreatment from responses to the medical school graduation questionnaire. Acad Med. 2014;89:705–11.
8. Kassebaum D, Culer E. On the culture of student abuse in medical school. Acad Med. 1998;73:1149–58.
9. National Patient Safety Foundation. Unmet needs: teaching physicians to provide safe patient care. Boston: Lucian Leape Institute at the National Patient Safety Foundation; 2010.
10. Cook AF, Arora VM, Rasinski KA, Curlin FA, Yoon JD. The prevalence of medical student mistreatment and its association with burnout. Acad Med. 2014;89:749–54.
11. Chadaga AR, Villines D, Krikorian A. Bullying in the American graduate medical education system: a national cross-sectional survey. PLoS One. 2016;11:e0150246.
12. Bahji A, Altomare J. Prevalence of intimidation, harassment, and discrimination among resident physicians: a systematic review and meta-analysis. Can Med Educ J. 2020;11:e97–e123.

13. Summary of HCAHPS survey results: January 2018 to December 2018 discharges. Centers for Medicare & Medicaid Services, 2019. Accessed 9 July 2020, at https://hcahpsonline.org/globalassets/hcahps/summary-analyses/summary-results/october-2019-public-report-january-2018%2D%2Ddecember-2018-discharges.pdf.

14. Leape LL. Unpublished Work.

15. Leape L, Fromson JA. Problem doctors: is there a system-level solution? Ann Intern Med. 2006;144:107–15.

16. Berge KH, Seppala MD, Schipper AM. Chemical dependency and the physician. Mayo Clin Proc. 2009;84:625–31.

17. Shanafelt TD, Hasan O, Dyrbye LN, et al. Changes in burnout and satisfaction with work-life balance in physicians and the general US working population between 2011 and 2014. Mayo Clin Proc. 2015;90:1600–13.

18. ABIM Foundation, American Board of Internal Medicine, ACP-ASIM Foundation, American College of Physicians-American Society of Internal Medicine, European Federation of Internal Medicine. Medical professionalism in the new millennium: a physician charter. Ann Intern Med. 2002;136:243–6.

19. Board certification: a trusted credential based on core competencies. American Board of Medical Specialties, [Archived February 15, 2020]. Accessed 9 July 2020, at https://web.archive.org/web/20200215154456/https:/www.abms.org/board-certification/a-trusted-credential/based-on-core-competencies.

20. Iglehart JK, Baron RB. Ensuring physicians' competence--is maintenance of certification the answer? N Engl J Med. 2012;367:2543–9.

21. Nasca TJ, Weiss KB, Bagian JP, Brigham TP. The accreditation system after the "next accreditation system". Acad Med. 2014;89:27–9.

22. Thompson CW. Medical boards let physicians practice despite drug abuse. The Washington Post; April 10, 2005.

23. National Practitioner Data Bank. https://www.npdb.hrsa.gov/index.jsp.

24. Federation of State Medical Boards Public Policy Compendium. Federation of State Medical Boards; 2007.

25. Federation of State Medical Boards Public Policy Compendium, policy 250.004 maintenance of licensure: Federation of State Medical Boards; 2011.

26. Thompson JN, Robin LA. State medical boards. J Legal Med. 2012;33:93–114.

27. Directory of physician assessment and remedial education programs. Federation of State Medical Boards. 2020. Accessed 9 July 2020, at https://www.fsmb.org/siteassets/spex/pdfs/remedprog.pdf.

28. Physician Assessment and Clinical Education (PACE). UC San Diego School of Medicine. Accessed 9 July 2020, at http://paceprogram.ucsd.edu/.

29. Chassin MR. Achieving and sustaining improved quality: lessons from New York state and cardiac surgery. Health Aff. 2002;21:40–51.

30. Leape LL, Hilborne LH, Park RE, et al. The appropriateness of use of coronary artery bypass graft surgery in New York state. JAMA. 1993;269:753–60.

31. Hilborne LH, Leape LL, Bernstein SJ, et al. The appropriateness of use of percutaneous transluminal coronary angioplasty in New York state. JAMA. 1993;269:761–5.
32. Bernstein SJ, Hilborne LH, Leape LL, et al. The appropriateness of use of coronary angiography in New York state. JAMA. 1993;269:766–70.
33. Localio AR, Lawthers AG, Brennan TA, et al. Relation between malpractice claims and adverse events due to negligence. N Engl J Med. 1991;325:245–51.
34. Cohen TH. Medical malpractice trials and verdicts in large counties, 2001. Washington, DC: Bureau of Justice Statistics; April 18, 2004.
35. Focused Professional Practice Evaluation (FPPE) - Understanding the requirements. The Joint Commission. Accessed 27 Sept 2020, at https://www.jointcommission.org/standards/standard-faqs/critical-access-hospital/medical-staff-ms/000001485/.
36. Lockyer J. Multisource feedback in the assessment of physician competencies. J Contin Educ Health Prof. 2003;23:4–12.
37. Donnon T, Al Ansari A, Al Alawi S, Violato C. The reliability, validity, and feasibility of multisource feedback physician assessment: a systematic review. Acad Med. 2014;89:511–6.
38. PULSE Program. Physicians Development Program Inc. Accessed 9 July 2020, at https://pulseprogram.com/.
39. Khuri SF, Daley J, Henderson WG. The comparative assessment and improvement of quality of surgical care in the Department of Veterans Affairs. Arch Surg. 2002;137:20–7.
40. Khuri SF, Daley J, Henderson W, et al. The Department of Veterans Affairs' NSQIP: the first national, validated, outcome-based, risk-adjusted, and peer-controlled program for the measurement and enhancement of the quality of surgical care. National VA Surgical Quality Improvement Program. Ann Surg. 1998;228:491–507.
41. ACS NSQIP Hospitals. The American College of Surgeons. Accessed 22 June 2020, at https://www.facs.org/search/nsqip-participants?allresults=.
42. Fink AS, Campbell DA Jr, Mentzer RM Jr, et al. The National Surgical Quality Improvement Program in non-veterans administration hospitals: initial demonstration of feasibility. Ann Surg. 2002;236:344–53.
43. Khuri SF. The NSQIP: a new frontier in surgery. Surgery. 2005;138:837–43.
44. Annandale E, Hunt K. Accounts of disagreements with doctors. Soc Sci Med. 1998;46:119–29.
45. Hickson GB, Federspiel CF, Pichert JW, Miller CS, Gauld-Jaeger J, Bost P. Patient complaints and malpractice risk. JAMA. 2002;287:2951–7.
46. Hickson GB, Pichert JW, Webb LE, Gabbe SG. A complementary approach to promoting professionalism: identifying, measuring, and addressing unprofessional behaviors. Acad Med. 2007;82:1040–8.
47. Vanderbilt Comprehensive Assessment Program. Vanderbilt University Medical Center. Accessed 9 July 2020, at https://www.vanderbilthealth.com/v-cap/.

48. Coalition for Physician Accountability. Accessed 9 July 2020, at http://www. physicianaccountability.org/.

49. Leape LL. Translating medical science into medical practice: do we need a national medical standards board? JAMA. 1995;273:1534–8.

50. Holmboe ES, Edgar L, Hamstra S. The milestones guidebook. Chicago: ACGME; 2016.

21

A Culture of Respect in Medicine

"The doctor treats me like an idiot." "He doesn't like people who ask questions." "He makes me feel like I'm wasting his time." (from a patient)

"When did you get your MD degree?" "When I want your advice, I'll ask for it." (doctor to a nurse)

"Is that what they teach you in medical school these days?" "Don't you know anything about renal anatomy?" (doctor to a medical student)

What is this all about? How can the noblest of professions, made up of intelligent, hard-working, dedicated people, have within its ranks some who treat others badly in their time of need? Why doesn't "professionalism" for all health-care professionals extend to ensuring that they live up to standards of decency and civility? As we have seen in the previous chapter, the reasons are complex, and disrespectful behavior is but one of many potential failings that doctors may suffer. But its influence is profound.

As the patient safety movement entered its second decade, experience with attempts to change systems led safety leaders to recognize that major progress could not occur without a supportive culture. And it became apparent that the major barrier to creating that culture, the core of the problem, was inappropriate physician behavior. This was, of course, the focus of our work on disclosure and apology: getting physicians to respect the patient's need for, and right to, full information on what went wrong when they were harmed by their care.

Physician behavior was also the focus of the attempts to reform medical education. The first LLI white paper, *Unmet Needs: Teaching physicians to provide safe patient care*, documented the alarming frequency of demeaning and dehumanizing treatment by faculty that medical students experienced. It came down with a strong recommendation that medical school deans and teaching hospital CEOs adopt a zero-tolerance policy for disrespectful or abusive behavior [1].

What is the patient experience? In my course on quality and patient safety at the Harvard School of Public Health, I collected disturbing data about the patient experience from my graduate students. Each year, at the beginning of the course, to ground their approach to quality improvement in real-world experience, I asked students to interview someone who had a serious medical problem. The students were to ask just two questions: What is it like living with this condition? What has been your experience with medical care? Consistently, over 10 years, nearly half of patients recounted episodes where they were treated in a demeaning or disrespectful way by their doctors, leaving memories that were often still vivid years later.

Even more than patients and students, nurses are on the receiving end of disrespectful treatment by physicians. Almost all nurses can tell stories of disruptive behavior and humiliation. Most of the physicians they work with treat them well, but it occurs frequently enough to poison the atmosphere and cause some to leave nursing.

Although available evidence does indicate that the percentage of doctors who engage in grossly disruptive behavior is small, many more engage in less flagrant types of disrespectful behavior. Dismissive put-downs of patients and nurses and "education by humiliation" or "pimping" of students are widely experienced. This had to change if we were to create the learning and supportive culture that is essential to safety. I became convinced that pervasive disrespect was the core of the culture problem. What could we do about it?

A Group of Leaders

Perhaps if Harvard took the lead, others would follow. If our staid, old, conservative hospitals could come to grips with the problem, others could as well. I raised the question to a number of knowledgeable, respected leaders who I knew at Harvard Medical School (HMS) and its hospitals. To my delight, but not surprise, they were all interested in taking it on. They knew disrespectful conduct was a serious problem, and they responded to the opportunity to do something about it.

In September 2010, I brought them together for dinner at the Harvard Faculty Club for the first meeting:

- *Ron Arky*, Professor of Medicine
- *Jules Dienstag*, Dean for Medical Education
- *Susan Edgman-Levitan*, Executive Director, Stoeckle Center, MGH
- *Dan Federman*, former Dean for Medical Education
- *Ed Hundert*, Director, Center for Teaching and Learning
- *Jeannette Ives-Erickson*, Vice President for Nursing, MGH
- *Gerry Healy*, Professor of Otology and Laryngology
- *Bob Mayer*, Professor of Medicine
- *Gregg Meyer*, Senior Vice President for Quality and Safety, MGH
- *Miles Shore*, Bullard Professor of Psychiatry and Chair, HMS Promotions and Review Board
- *Richard Schwartzstein*, Professor of Medicine, Director of the Academy, HMS
- *Andy Whittemore*, Professor of Surgery and Chief Medical Officer, BWH

I welcomed the group with a blunt statement that the purpose of the meeting was not to *talk* about unprofessional behavior, but to determine if we wanted to *do* something about it. I laid out the scope: disruptive behavior, humiliation of students and nurses, disrespectful treatment of patients, and passive resistance and non-participation in quality improvement. I gave them statistics from surveys of nurses and medical students and read quotes from my students' papers describing episodes of dismissive and demeaning treatment of patients by their doctors.

A great discussion followed: we tolerate disrespect, it is a leadership issue, reform has to come from the top; we have actually rewarded bad behavior, we need a system to deal with it, we should do "360" evaluations of everyone, etc. Members recounted examples of bad conduct and poor support of students and nurses; it was more than just a problem of individual professionalism, as so often described, it was the culture.

We agreed that it was time for action and that a statement from HMS would be powerful. We would meet again.

At the second meeting, we found broad agreement that the problem was severe and prevalent, that leadership is necessary to address the issue, and that we needed a different structure for responding to bad behavior. Our goal would be to develop an institution-wide (all HMS teaching hospitals) program. We would identify structures and processes that need to be put in place to identify and deal with disrespectful conduct of all kinds: i.e., the specifics of what we wanted hospitals to do. We decided to write a white paper laying out the problem and our recommendations and try to get HMS leadership and hospital CEOs on board.

"Champions"

I also convened a second group: frontline safety leaders at each of the teaching hospitals who could advise us on implementation. I dubbed this group of key safety people "Champions" from our QI jargon, i.e., clinical leaders who make things happen. I saw the two groups as symbiotic: the senior, professionalism working group would develop theory and policy, and the frontline leaders would work on the ground-level implementation.

This Champions group, all of whom I knew, and all physicians, included:

- *Bob Truog*, Children's Hospital
- *Sigall Bell*, Beth Israel Deaconess Hospital
- *John Herman*, Mass General Hospital
- *Craig Bunnell*, Dana-Farber Cancer Institute
- *Jo Shapiro*, Brigham and Women's Hospital
- *Elizabeth Gaufberg*, Cambridge Health Alliance
- *Mitch Rein*, North Shore Hospital
- *Les Selbovitz*, Newton Wellesley Hospital
- *Susan Abookire*, Mt Auburn Hospital
- *Luke Sato*, CRICO

As with the senior group, all were eager to participate. I explained the different functions of the two groups: the senior group's mission was to motivate the Dean and the hospital CEOs to develop and implement more effective policies and processes for dealing with disrespectful behavior; we were writing a white paper for that. The Champions' group would develop strategies and plans for implementation. An obvious place for them to start was the current situation regarding codes of conduct. So, in preparation for the first meeting, I asked each of them to send me their hospital's code for dealing with disrespectful behavior.

The Champions first convened in January. The codes were all over the map! Several hospitals didn't even have a code! I thought this would be a great opportunity: we could work together to come up with a universal code that all Harvard hospitals could agree to.

But the group had little interest in that. They weren't sure just what they were interested in, but my various suggestions fell on deaf ears. We spent the first meeting with each person talking about what they were doing in their institutions and agreed to meet again. We met several times over the next year but could never really agree on proceeding in a clear direction. To my great disappointment, in the end the group had no positive impact. But, as we shall see, it did have an unfortunate negative effect.

Meanwhile, the senior working group met monthly over the period of a year and were very active. We wanted the medical school to take the lead here, but that would not be easy. Because of the unusual structure of HMS in which all of the teaching hospitals are fairly autonomous, the Dean was sensitive to their strong sense of independence and not anxious to tell them what to do. We gathered information on codes and practices and outlined the paper. We added several people to the group: deans Maureen Connelly and Gretchen Brodnicki; the Chairman of Faculty Discipline, Paul Russell; and Luke Sato from CRICO, our liability insurer.

Miles Shore and I went to work drafting a white paper that would lay out the various aspects of disrespect, defining the types of behavior and the varied situations where it occurred. We had learned a great deal from our research; the problem was far worse than we had suspected. There was ample evidence: studies documenting the extent to which nurses, students, and doctors were treated badly, plus the trove of patient stories from my students' interviews.

The Problem

Disruptive behavior was what brought us together, and it was the situation crying out most loudly for solution. As noted, most nurses experience shouting, demeaning comments, or humiliation by a physician at some time, many frequently. Similarly, while most of their encounters with physicians are positive, many patients have had a bad experience. Almost all medical students can recount humiliating treatment by their teaching attendings in hospitals.

The most disturbing finding from our review of the literature and pooled experience, however, was not about disruptive behavior, but that lesser types of disrespectful behavior are pervasive and not limited to physicians. While only a few "bad apples" engaged in obvious egregious disruptive behavior, lesser degrees of disrespectful conduct were common.

Passive aggressive behavior is a pervasive form of disrespect, but it is seldom commented on. For example, many physicians have not been enthusiastic about patient safety—they claim to not see the problem in their own practices, and they are too busy to participate in hospital-organized "quality improvement" projects. When asked or required to participate, they act out their resistance passively—by missing or coming late to meetings, by not offering ideas or doing the work, by being slow to carry out their tasks.

Another pervasive aspect of disrespect that is not even recognized by those affected is systemic or *institutionalized* disrespect. This is the disrespect embedded in many of the well-accepted practices that are part of everyday care in hospitals. The most obvious example is working conditions. Research evidence is clear that long hours, sleep deprivation, and excessive workloads cause increased errors. Yet, long hours and heavy workloads are standard operating procedures in health care, especially in teaching hospitals.

If you stop and think about it, requiring doctors and nurses to work under these conditions is the ultimate in disrespect. Not only are you treating them badly, you are *knowingly* putting them in a position where they are more likely to harm their patients. For hospital leaders, administrative or clinical, to do so is unconscionable, yet it is the norm almost everywhere.

A more subtle form of institutionalized disrespect is waiting times. Millions of hours are lost every day in the USA by patients waiting for care. We say, in effect, your time is worth less than my time. We ignore the immense costs, social and fiscal, of keeping people out of work and children out of school. Patients bear the brunt of this form of disrespect, but the inefficiency also exacts its toll from the physicians and employees who also wait.

And it is unnecessary. Operational research has developed methods for "queuing" and task management that virtually eliminate waiting and are well-known; they just need to be implemented. Some hospitals have done that and even eliminated waiting rooms [2]. All hospitals and doctors' offices should.

The evidence of pervasive disrespect in health care is clear, but the literature was remarkably shy of insight into the *causes* of disrespect. For this we had to rely on the insights about general human behavior gathered over the years by psychologists. We did find examples of some very well-thought-out policies and procedures for dealing with egregious behavior, particularly the College of Physicians and Surgeons of Ontario's *Guidebook for Managing Disruptive Physician Behavior* [3].

A Culture of Respect

By March we had completed a first draft, and various members were working on revisions. Jeff Flier, Dean of HMS, had indicated that he would welcome a proposal for a policy on respectful behavior. However, in the end he preferred that we distribute the white paper to Harvard hospitals and not to colleagues on the quad, the formal HMS campus.

The group thought it should also be published in the medical literature, so Miles Shore and I worked with several other members to finish the paper, and in July 2011 we submitted it to Academic Medicine. I was dubious that such a long paper would be published by a journal. Fortunately, the editor recognized its value and accepted it with the proviso that we break it into two papers that were published in the same issue:

A Culture of Respect, Part 1: The Nature and Causes of Disrespectful Behavior by Physicians [4]

The first paper described the dimensions and the extent of the problem of disrespectful behavior.

The numbers are arresting: 95% of nurses have witnessed or received abuse, and 64% reported an episode of verbal abuse at least every 2–3 months. But the number of doctors responsible is small: 5.7% [5]. More than a third of nurses believe disruptive behavior is a cause of nurses leaving an institution [6].

As noted in Chap. 20, abuse of medical students is also common. Dismissive comments or humiliation is experienced by two thirds of students [1, 7, 8]. More than half show signs of burnout, and 14% have symptoms of serious depression. Half of residents are victims of bullying, belittling, and humiliation [9]. Patient surveys show that 13–27% of patients report problems with doctor communication [10]. Patient interviews show the percentage is closer to 50% [11].

The paper then defined the types of disrespectful behavior and their effects and explored the causes of disrespect. We proposed that the slow progress in patient safety results from the dysfunctional culture of health-care institutions, and the root cause of that dysfunctional culture is disrespectful behavior.

Six different forms of disrespect were identified as common in health-care organizations:

1. *Disruptive behavior*, such as angry outbursts, threats, bullying, and the use of profane and abusive language
2. *Humiliating and demeaning treatment of nurses, residents, and students*
3. *Passive-aggressive behavior*, such as blaming others for your failures and making frequent negative comments about the hospital or colleagues
4. *Passive disrespect*, such as being chronically late to meetings, delay in dictating charts, and resistance to following safe practices, such as hand washing
5. *Dismissive treatment of patients*

6. *Systemic disrespect*: practices that are taken for granted, such as long hours and excessive workloads for nurses and residents, long waiting times for patients, and not disclosing and apologizing after harm caused by an error

All of these forms of disrespect create barriers to communication among all parties—doctors, nurses, residents, and patients. Disrespect is a major barrier to efforts to improve patient safety. It undermines the teamwork that is essential to changing systems to improve safety; it saps meaning and satisfaction from work, leading to burnout and low morale. It is particularly damaging to students and patients, especially when they are harmed by a medical error.

We identified both internal (individual) and external (environmental) causes of disrespectful behavior. Internal causes include personal feelings of insecurity and anxiety, depression, narcissism, aggressiveness, and prior victimization. The extent to which these antecedent problems result in disrespectful behavior, however, is largely determined by the external environment.

Key environmental factors that foster disrespect are the hierarchical nature of health-care organizations and a blaming culture. But also important are the long hours, heavy workloads, and "production pressure" to deliver quality care.

A Culture of Respect, Part 2: Creating a Culture of Respect [12]

The main theme of the second paper is that creating a culture of respect is the core of the broader cultural transformation that is needed to create a culture of safety in health care. The responsibility for creating a culture of respect falls squarely on the shoulders of the organization's leader "because only he or she can set the tone and initiate the processes that lead to change."

We challenged health-care organization CEOs to accomplish five major tasks:

1. *To motivate and inspire* others to take action "and to create a sense of urgency around doing so"

2. *To establish preconditions for a culture of respect* by showing concern for the well-being of faculty and staff by addressing issues of hours and workloads and physical hazards
3. To *establish policies regarding disrespectful behavior,* i.e., *codes of conduct*
4. To *facilitate engagement of frontline workers* by addressing systemic stressors
5. To *create a learning environment* by modeling professional behavior and valuing the learner

The paper then provided extensive and explicit recommendations on creating a code of conduct, drawing on experience from various sources, especially the College of Physicians and Surgeons of Ontario's *Guidebook for Managing Disruptive Physician Behavior* [13]. We emphasized the importance of developing effective means of implementing and enforcing such a code, including enabling safe reporting and responding promptly.

The final section dealt with prevention, which includes education at all levels, the design and use of appropriate performance evaluations, and support of individuals at all levels who work to create a safe environment. Creating transparency, breaking down authoritarianism, learning to work in teams, and creating a "just culture" are all part of the challenge of creating a respectful culture.

A Strange Twist

When we submitted the papers to Academic Medicine in July 2011, I sent a copy to each member of the Champions group knowing they would be interested in what we had learned. To my great surprise, several were upset that they hadn't been included as authors! I thought this was a bit weird, because 6 months earlier I had sent them a draft so they would know what we were doing (presumably the foundation for their work), and we discussed the findings at a Champions meeting. Only one person sent me any comments about it, and no one suggested any edits. Given this prior behavior, it was a mystery to me why any of them would now think they were entitled to authorship.

Clearly, however, there was a major miscommunication that even in retrospect neither Miles nor I nor any of the authors were able to understand. We spent a great deal of time trying to mollify the Champions and resolve differences. Several disagreed substantially with the emphasis of the paper on consequences and response rather than on a supportive culture. They were upset about being left out of a major paper on this subject coming from Harvard—despite the fact they had contributed nothing to it!

Meanwhile, the paper was provisionally accepted, with the usual request that we respond to reviewers' comments. We saw this as an opportunity to ask several of the disaffected to write an additional section in response to the reviewers, in which they could weave in some of their ideas and be legitimately added as authors. I thought this was a good solution.

However, despite the general angst, only two of them volunteered to do this. Unfortunately, instead of writing an additional section, they set about rewriting the whole paper! This would obviously not be acceptable to the editors, but they were insistent. So the whole effort ended in naught. I felt very bad about it—especially since a number of the group were old friends and associates.

Response

The two papers came out in the Annals of Internal Medicine in July 2012 and were well received. The earliest most obvious impact in our hospitals was that several tightened up their procedures and fired some of their most outrageous offenders, physicians whom colleagues had complained about for years.

A more impressive tangible result was that Virginia Mason Medical Center (VMMC) took the papers to heart. Nationally recognized as the leader in reducing errors and creating a culture of safety, VMMC was a fertile field in which this seed could germinate. Not only did VMMC upgrade their standards and processes for dealing with disrespectful behavior, they developed a comprehensive continuing education course on respect and required all 5000 of their staff and employees to take it. The course has subsequently been marketed to hundreds of other hospitals worldwide.

It is hard to measure the impact of the papers nationally, but I noticed that the word "respect" began to appear in conversations and writings about quality and safety. More specifically, medical schools and residency programs now routinely survey students and residents about receiving abusive behavior. Questions about how their doctors treated them were added to the post- hospitalization questionnaires that were sent to patients to evaluate their care. The feedback from those surveys puts immense pressure on hospitals, which, perhaps more than anything else, is slowly leading to a more respectful environment.

References

1. National Patient Safety Foundation. Unmet needs: teaching physicians to provide safe patient care. Boston: Lucian Leape Institute at the National Patient Safety Foundation; 2010.
2. Kenney C. Transforming health care: the Virginia Mason Medical Center story. New York: Wiley; 2011.
3. Barer ML, Evans RG, Stoddart GL. Controlling health care costs by direct charges to patients. Toronto: Ontario Economic Council; 1979.
4. Leape L, Shore M, Dienstag J, et al. A culture of respect: I. The nature and causes of disrespectful behavior. Acad Med. 2012;87:845–52.
5. Rosenstein AH, O'Daniel M. A survey of the impact of disruptive behaviors and communication defects on patient safety. Jt Comm J Qual Patient Saf. 2008;34:464–71.
6. Rosenstein AH, Russell H, Lauve R. Disruptive physician behavior contributes to nursing shortage. Study links bad behavior by doctors to nurses leaving the profession. Physician Exec. 2002;28:8–11.
7. Leape L, Fromson JA. Problem doctors: is there a system-level solution? Ann Intern Med. 2006;144:107–15.
8. Kassebaum D, Culer E. On the culture of student abuse in medical school. Acad Med. 1998;73:1149–58.
9. Chadaga AR, Villines D, Krikorian A. Bullying in the American graduate medical education system: a national cross-sectional survey. PLoS One. 2016;11:e0150246.
10. HCAHPS fact sheet (CAHPS hospital survey). AHRQ; 2010. Accessed 29 Mar 2012, at http://www.hcahpsonline.org/files/HCAHPS%20Fact%20 Sheet%202010.pdf.

11. Leape LL. Unpublished data.
12. Leape L, Shore M, Dienstag J, et al. A culture of respect, part 2: creating a culture of respect. Acad Med. 2012;87:853–8.
13. Ontario_College_of_Physicians_and_Surgeons. Guidebook for managing disruptive physician behavior. Toronto; 2008.

Part IV
Building a Culture of Patient Safety

22

Making Plans for the Road Ahead

Despite encouraging progress in the early years of the patient safety movement, it soon became evident that there were deeper issues that needed to be addressed. We realized that we were not going to make health care safe by making process changes one by one, even powerful changes such as eliminating CLABSI or implementing the surgical checklist.

We needed to fundamentally reimagine the way we think about delivery of health care. Health care needed not just to be improved but to be transformed. A sustainable strategy—probably several strategies—was needed to enable us to deal with the fundamental systemic and behavioral issues that drive unsafe behavior.

Fortunately, as noted in Chap. 5, in 2007 the National Patient Safety Foundation created a mechanism to do that, the *Lucian Leape Institute*, a "think tank" of experts whose leadership roles had given them experience and insights that would enable them to identify the issues and make authoritative recommendations for changes.

The charge to the Institute was to "define strategic paths and calls to action for the field of patient safety and provide vision and context for the many efforts underway within the health care system. Through its Roundtables, it will issue reports that will guide the work of the field and challenge the system to address the issues critical to making the system safer."

I chaired the Institute. The other initial members were:

- *Don Berwick*, founder and CEO of the Institute for Healthcare Improvement, who brought quality improvement to health care
- *Carolyn Clancy*, Director, Agency for Healthcare Research and Quality, who spearheaded its early work on safety
- *Jim Conway*, Senior VP, Institute for Healthcare Improvement and previous COO of Dana-Farber Cancer Institute, who led its reorganization for safety
- *David Lawrence*, CEO of Kaiser Foundation Health Plan, former Executive Session member, who brought patient safety to Kaiser-Permanente
- *Julianne Morath*, Chief Quality and Safety Officer, Vanderbilt University Medical Center, who led Allina Health's entry into patient safety
- *Dennis O'Leary*, President of the Joint Commission, also a former Executive Session member, who focused the Commission on patient safety
- *Paul Gluck*, immediate past chair of NPSF Board of Directors
- *Diane Pinakiewicz*, President of NPSF

At the first meeting of the Lucian Leape Institute, we had a lively discussion about our purpose and how to most effectively go about strategic planning. After surfacing dozens of ideas, we decided to focus our efforts on core concepts that we believed were foundational to achieving meaningful improvement in patient safety.

They were obviously not the *only* thing needed, but we believed they were essential. Without embracing these concepts, health-care

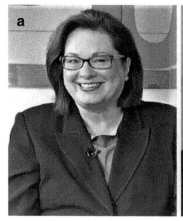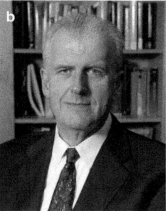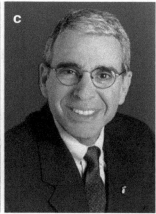

(**a**) Julie Morath, (**b**) Jim Conway, and (**c**) Paul Gluck.

organizations could not mobilize the resources and motivate their workforce to achieve safe care. We identified five concepts: Reforming Medical Education, Integrating Care, Finding Joy and Meaning in Work, Patient Engagement, and Transparency. We called them *Transforming Concepts*.

Each concept requires a change of consciousness to move thinking beyond traditional boundaries, and each implies profound behavioral changes. We wrote a paper, *Transforming health care: a safety imperative*, that explained the transforming concepts, summarized the importance of each, and defined the issues to be resolved [1]. Then we set to work.

Over the next several years, LLI convened a roundtable of national experts and stakeholders, including patient advocates, for each of the five concepts to explore the critical issues, understand them better, and make recommendations for transformative change. To stimulate buy-in and ownership, we made a special effort to include on each panel leaders of organizations for which the issue was especially relevant and who could implement the recommendations. LLI members chaired the roundtables.

The typical roundtable had 25–30 participants and met twice in two-day sessions. We had no trouble recruiting members for each topic; the relevant thought leaders shared our interest and were eager to participate. Prior to convening, we provided participants with a comprehensive literature review on the topic. The discussions were spirited and wide-ranging and concluded with recommendations for health-care organizations and their leaders.

Following each roundtable, the leaders wrote a white paper that combined facts and insights from the literature with the results of the panel discussions to provide a comprehensive account of the topic with specific recommendations for action by health-care providers, leaders, and policy makers. These white papers are available, free of charge from IHI at IHI.org.

The five white papers are summarized below, including for each also a review of progress made since the paper was published and a discussion of remaining challenges. These are verbatim combinations of text taken from two summaries later published by LLI: *Transforming Health Care: A Compendium of Reports from the National Patient Safety Foundation's Lucian Leape Institute*, IHI, 2016 [2], and *Transforming concepts in patient safety: a progress report.* BMJ Quality & Safety, 2018 [3].

Unmet Needs [4]

Teaching Physicians to Provide Safe Patient Care

Workshop Leaders: Dennis O'Leary and Lucian Leape

Health-care delivery continues to be unsafe despite major patient safety improvement efforts over the past decade. The roundtable concluded that substantive improvements in patient safety will be difficult to achieve without major medical education reform at the medical school and residency training program levels. Medical schools must assure that future physicians not only have the requisite knowledge, skills, behaviors, and attitudes to practice competently but also are prepared to play active roles in identifying and resolving patient safety problems. These competencies should become fully developed during the residency training period.

Medical schools today focus principally on providing students with the knowledge and skills they need for the technical practice of medicine but often pay inadequate attention to the shaping of student skills, attitudes, and behaviors that will permit them to function safely and as architects of patient safety improvement in the future. Specifically, medical schools are not doing an adequate job of facilitating student understanding of basic knowledge and the development of skills required for the provision of safe patient care, to wit: systems thinking, problem analysis, application of human factors science, communication skills, patient-centered care, teaming concepts and skills, and dealing with feelings of doubt, fear, and uncertainty with respect to medical errors.

In addition, medical students all too often suffer demeaning experiences at the hands of faculty and residents, a phenomenon that appears to reflect serious shortcomings in the medical school and teaching hospital cultures. Behaviors like these that are disruptive to professional relationships have adverse effects upon students, residents, nurses, colleagues, and even patients. Students frequently tend to emulate these behaviors as they become residents and practicing clinicians, which perpetuates work environments and cultures that are antithetical to the delivery of safe, patient-centered care.

Summary of Recommendations (Table 22.1)

Table 22.1 Key recommendations from *Unmet Needs: Teaching Physicians to Provide Safe Patient Care*

Target of recommendation	Recommendation
Medical school and hospital leaders	Place the highest priority on creating a learning culture that emphasizes patient safety, professionalism, transparency, and valuing the individual learner
	Eliminate hierarchical and authority gradients
	Emphasize that professionalism includes demonstrating mutual respect and non-tolerance of abusive or demeaning behavior
	Declare and enforce a zero-tolerance policy for confirmed egregious disrespectful behavior by faculty, staff, or residents
	Promote the development of interpersonal skills, leadership, teamwork, and collaboration among faculty and staff
	Provide incentives and resources to enhance faculty capabilities to teach and practice patient safety and to be effective role models
	The selection process for admission to medical schools should emphasize attributes that reflect professionalism and orientation to patient safety, such as compassion, empathy, and collaboration
Medical schools	Treat patient safety as a science that encompasses human factors, systems theory, and open communication
	Emphasize the shaping of desired skills, attitudes, and behaviors as set forth in the core competencies defined by the IOM, the American Board of Medical Specialties, and the Accreditation Council for Graduate Medical Education
	The educational experience should be coherent, continuing, and flexible throughout undergraduate medical education, residency and fellowship training, and lifelong continuing education
Accrediting bodies	Amend medical school accreditation requirements and residency program requirements to include expectations for the creation of learning cultures and the development of patient safety-related behavioral traits.
	Survey medical schools to evaluate education priorities for patient safety and the creation of school and hospital cultures that support patient safety

Progress

In recent years, medical school curricula have increasingly included patient safety and safety science, and these concepts have also become more common in education for other clinicians and frontline staff. For example, the American Medical Association's Accelerating Change in Medical Education Consortium brought medical schools together to innovate, develop curricula, and share best practices, including those addressing quality and safety.

The Accreditation Council for Graduate Medical Education Clinical Learning Environment Review (ACGME CLER) program requires medical resident participation in quality and safety learning. Recently, the Association of American Medical Colleges (AAMC) initiated a program to create a shared understanding of Quality Improvement and Patient Safety (QIPS) competencies across the full continuum from medical school to continuing practice.

Other clinical disciplines, particularly nursing, have often pioneered educational pathways, and a concerted effort is underway to emphasize the importance of interprofessional teams. The Quality and Safety Education for Nurses (QSEN) program has focused on enhancing education around safety science in nursing schools for more than a decade. More recently, the National Collaborative for Improving the Clinical Learning Environment (NCICLE) highlighted the "patient safety gap" in the education and training of all clinicians and provided clear recommendations for improvement [3].

To assist health-care students and professionals in building core skills in improvement, safety, and leadership, the Institute for Healthcare Improvement (IHI) developed a web-based interactive educational program called the Open School. More than 650,000 learners have enrolled in the Open School since it opened its virtual doors in 2008.

To address the need for training in postgraduate medical education, in 2012 the NPSF created a course in patient safety and safety science that more than 7000 learners of diverse disciplines have utilized. Several universities have developed graduate education and fellowships in quality and safety, and clinicians, risk managers, pharmacists, executives, and others have pursued these as well as certificate programs and professional certification in patient safety.

Remaining Challenges

Still, opportunity lies ahead for greater consistency in how health professionals learn about patient safety. A 2016 report from ACGME CLER reveals gaps in areas such as feedback on safety reporting and experiential learning, lack of awareness of the range of patient safety issues, and shortage of opportunities for interprofessional system-based improvement efforts. Contributing to this learning gap is a shortage of academic faculty with safety and quality improvement expertise.

Continuing education requirements for attending physicians are highly variable. While some medical specialties require continuing education in patient safety, the American Board of Internal Medicine recently removed it as a requirement from Maintenance of Certification. Health-care organizations would benefit from encouraging study of safety science by all team members, including board members, and operationalizing ways to achieve continuous learning as safety science expands.

As these and other activities gain momentum, the core agenda remains consistent, clear, and urgent: to mainstream the preparation of health professionals' awareness, skills, commitment, and practical training about the scientific pursuit of safer care. Embracing the science of safety in medical education is crucial to the future health and well-being of patients, families, and communities.

Order from Chaos [5]

Accelerating Care Integration

Workshop Leaders: David Lawrence and Richard Bohmer

Lack of care coordination and integration was identified as a major contributor to the frequency of avoidable errors in patient care in the Institute of Medicine (IOM) report *To Err Is Human* (1999). Care integration was presented as the cornerstone for achieving high quality in the subsequent IOM report *Crossing the Quality Chasm* (2001). The Agency for Healthcare Research and Quality (AHRQ) has included care integration and patient safety in its scope of work since early in this decade. Federal government administration arguments for the Patient Protection and Affordable Care Act of 2010 included numerous references to this issue.

Modern care delivery is extraordinarily complex. To protect the patient and avoid errors require a planned, coordinated, and fully integrated approach to care. In addition to the complexity inherent in modern treatment for patients with difficult and often multiple conditions, complexity is found throughout the care experience: in the number of physicians involved, the number of professionals and support personnel required, the multiple venues where care is provided, and the diverse requirements and expectations of patients. As a consequence, the risks of harm also rise unless careful attention is given to the way care is organized and delivered, that is, to the system of care delivery itself. The system must be designed to protect the patient while ensuring that he or she receives the full benefits of the remarkable advances that have occurred over the past century.

And here we arrive at care integration, the planned, thoughtful design of the care process for the benefit and protection of the patient. Unfortunately, physicians and leaders of delivery systems (with notable exceptions such as those at the Mayo Clinic, Geisinger Health System, and Kaiser-Permanente) have been unwilling or unable to embrace greater care integration. As described in *Crossing the Quality Chasm*, most patient care is fragmented and uncoordinated. Where integration has occurred, it is most often structural: assembling piece parts under a single governance umbrella while leaving the underlying care delivery processes largely untouched.

The care delivery system is struggling to escape the straitjacket of physician autonomy and economic independence, a payment system that reinforces fragmentation and independent decision-making, and a regulatory framework that places legal responsibility on the individual professional without corresponding accountability of the team or the system within which that professional works. The medical education system reinforces these expectations and does little to prepare new physicians for the team-based, interdependent work that is required to achieve high-quality and safe care.

Summary of Recommendations (Table 22.2)

Table 22.2 Key recommendations from *Order from Chaos: Accelerating Care Integration*

Target of recommendation	Recommendation
All stakeholders: federal and state governmental agencies, consumer groups	Create mechanisms for developing a shared understanding among public and private stakeholders regarding the link between care integration and patient safety
	Utilize working groups and public forums, best practices, and patient stories to be catalogued and disseminated
Health-care leaders and practitioners, public	Patients and families must become active participants in process improvement and design and redesign efforts and review organizational performance
Regulatory and accrediting bodies	Create methods of measuring care integration, along with robust assessment and evaluation metrics, and incorporate these measures into public reporting systems
Medical schools, professional societies, nonprofits	Provide education and training for executives, boards, clinicians, and medical students that focus on patient safety and care integration
Researchers, industry	Develop the technology and infrastructure to allow for national spread of organizational and operational expertise to support care integration

Progress

With an increased call for improved coordination of care and focus on patient safety across the care continuum, methods for improving handoffs and communication among teams, providers, and patients are gaining traction. Today the focus on population health and market-specific shifts in payment models serve as incentives for greater care integration and coordination.

Progress has been made to develop systems and structures to encourage and incentivize care integration. Accountable care organizations (ACOs) have brought together groups of health providers to incentivize better quality care at a lower cost. Likewise, the development of the patient-centered medical home (PCMH) aims to reorganize and reinvigorate primary care, and early evidence shows promise in achieving lower costs, improved patient experience, and better care quality.

Other encouraging examples of improved care integration include Project Re-Engineered Discharge (Project RED), the PCORI-funded Project ACHIEVE (Achieving Patient-Centered Care and Optimized Health In Care Transitions by Evaluating the Value of Evidence), and the Johns Hopkins School of Nursing–led Community Aging in Place: Advancing Better Living for Elders (CAPABLE). For example, Project RED developed strategies to improve the hospital discharge process to promote patient safety and has been proven to reduce rehospitalizations and yield high rates of patient satisfaction.

Finally, the increase in employed physicians and continued refinement of the electronic health record have accelerated care integration. Improving interoperability of health information technology has been a major initiative at the federal level to improve information flow across the entire care continuum.

Remaining Challenges

Despite incremental improvement, coordination and integration of care remain difficult, particularly for patients with multiple chronic conditions. Even with a national push toward more integrated care models (perhaps most focused on the development of ACOs), so far results toward safer, more coordinated care have been mixed. Furthermore, care integration issues are compounded for older adults. One study found that the average Medicare beneficiary spent about 17 days in contact with the health-care system through an average of 3.4 different clinicians. Only 55% of these individuals coordinated their care principally with a single primary care physician.

Structural changes alone will not ensure optimal care integration. Strong clinician leadership and patient engagement will be required to further improve care coordination. Involving patients and families in the codesign of care, especially around coordination and care delivered in the home, will help identify unmet needs and educational deficits.

Care integration remains perhaps the most challenging of the transforming concepts because of the fragmentation of the US health-care system. When Americans are asked to reflect on the integration of care from their own experiences, some refer to the term "health-care system" as an oxymoron.

Individuals responsible for coordinating care and helping patients navigate the care system include primary care physicians, specialists, nurses, pharmacists, social workers, and care managers, as well as health plan and delivery system personnel. As care becomes more complex and shared among more providers, it is essential to improve both processes (e.g., teamwork, communication, and patient engagement) and technologies (e.g., EHRs) for patients and providers.

Through the Eyes of the Workforce [6]

Creating Joy, Meaning, and Safer Health Care

Workshop Leaders: Julie Morath and Paul O'Neill

The health-care workforce is composed of well-intentioned, well-prepared people in a variety of roles and clinical disciplines who do their best every day to ensure that patients are well cared for. It is from this mission of caring for people in times of their greatest vulnerability and need that health-care workers find meaning in their work, as well as their experience of joy.

Yet many health-care workers suffer harm—emotional and physical—in the course of providing care. Many are subjected to being bullied, harassed, demeaned, ignored, and, in the most extreme cases, physically assaulted. They are also physically injured by working in conditions of known and preventable environmental risk. In addition, production and cost pressures have reduced complex, intimate, caregiving relationships into a series of demanding tasks performed under severe time constraints. Under these conditions, it is difficult for caregivers to find purpose and joy in their work or to meet the challenge of making health care safe for patients they serve.

Vulnerable Workplaces

The basic precondition of a safe workplace is protection of the physical and psychological safety of the workforce. Both are conspicuously absent or considered optional in many care delivery organizations. The prevalence of physical harm experienced by the health-care workforce is striking, much higher than in other industries. Up to a third of nurses experience back or musculoskeletal injuries in a year, and many have unprotected contact with blood-borne pathogens.

Psychological harm is also common. In many health-care organizations, staff are not treated with respect—or, worse yet, they are routinely treated with disrespect. Emotional abuse, bullying, and even threats of physical assault and learning by humiliation are all often accepted as "normal" conditions of the health-care workplace, creating a culture of fear and intimidation that saps joy and meaning from work.

The absence of cultural norms that create the preconditions of psychological and physical safety obscures meaning of work and drains motivation. The costs of burnout, litigation, lost work hours, employee turnover, and the inability to attract newcomers to caring professions are wasteful and add to the burden of illness. Disrespectful treatment of workers increases the risk of patient injury.

What Can Be Done?

An environment of mutual respect is critical if the workforce is to find joy and meaning in work. In modern health care, teamwork is essential for safe practice, and teamwork is impossible in the absence of mutual respect.

Former CEO of Alcoa Paul O'Neill advises that, to find joy and meaning in their daily work, each person in the workforce must be able to answer affirmatively three questions each day:

1. Am I treated with dignity and respect by everyone?
2. Do I have what I need so I can make a contribution that gives meaning to my life?
3. Am I recognized and thanked for what I do?

Developing Effective Organizations

To create a safe and supportive work environment, health-care organizations must become effective, high-reliability organizations, characterized by continuous learning, improvement, teamwork, and transparency. Effective organizations care for their employees and continuously meet preconditions not subject to annual priority and budget setting. The most fundamental precondition is workforce safety, physical and psychological. The workforce needs to know that their safety is an enduring and non-negotiable priority for the governing board, CEO, and organization.

Knowing that their well-being is a priority enables the workforce to be meaningfully engaged in their work, to be more satisfied, less likely to experience burnout, and to deliver more effective and safer care.

Achieving this vision requires leadership. The governing board, CEO, and organizational leaders create the cultural norms and conditions that produce workforce safety, meaning, and joy. Effective leaders shape safety culture through management practices that demonstrate a priority to safety and compassionately engage the workforce to speak about and report errors, mistakes, and hazards that threaten safety—their own or their patients'. Joy and meaning will be created when the workforce feels valued, safe from harm, and part of the solutions for change.

Summary of Recommendations (Table 22.3)

Table 22.3 Key recommendations from *Through the Eyes of the Workforce: Creating Joy, Meaning, and Safer Health Care*

Target of recommendation	Recommendation
Hospital and health-care leaders, professionals, board members	Develop and embody shared core values of mutual respect and civility; transparency and truth telling; safety of all workers and patients; and alignment and accountability from the boardroom through the front lines
Hospital and health-care leaders, professionals, board members	Adopt the explicit aim to eliminate harm to workforce and patients
	Recognize and celebrate the work and accomplishments of the work force, regularly and with high visibility
Hospital and health-care leaders, board members, managers	Commit to creating a high-reliability organization (HRO) and demonstrate the discipline to achieve highly reliable performance This will require creating a learning and improvement system and adopting evidence-based management skills for reliability
Hospital and health-care leaders	Establish data capture, database, and performance metrics for improvement and accountability
Government and nonprofit funders	Support industry-wide research to explore issues and conditions in health care that are harming our workforce and patients

Progress

Multiple initiatives are underway to increase awareness of the importance of joy and meaning in work and workforce safety. The National Academy of Medicine and several health-care professional groups and insurers, such as the American Association of Critical-Care Nurses (AACN), the American Nurses Association (ANA Enterprise), the American Medical Association (AMA), and the Harvard Risk Management Foundation are addressing the issue of resilience and burnout.

IHI has developed a framework for increasing joy in work that recommends domains such as reward and recognition, choice and autonomy, camaraderie and teamwork, and physical and psychological safety. Some have observed that the widely accepted Triple Aim should be expanded to include workforce safety and joy and meaning in work—the Quadruple Aim.

Regarding health-care workforce physical safety, noteworthy efforts are proceeding. With the support of the Centers for Medicare & Medicaid Services (CMS), the US Occupational Safety and Health Administration recently launched an initiative to encourage hospitals and health-care facilities to implement safety and health management systems to prevent injuries among their workforce and patients. Similarly, the Joint Commission has provided detailed reports and tools for improving workforce safety and reducing workplace violence.

Remaining Challenges

Despite these efforts, according to one recent study, more than half of US physicians suffer from burnout. Among critical-care nurses, 25%–33% have symptoms of severe burnout syndrome. Not only do physicians have higher rates of burnout than the general public, but they also suffer higher rates of depression and suicide. The Covid pandemic has substantially increased all of these problems. The effects of psychological, emotional, and physical harm to the workforce surface in the form of litigation, lost work hours, employee turnover, and inability to attract newcomers to caring professions. With health-care reform, pay-for-performance, the introduction of electronic health records, and other innovations, health-care workers spend less time directly caring for patients—further draining energy, meaning, and joy.

Compounding the issue, a recent survey found that only 23% of hospital boards review workplace safety dashboards. Our health-care workforce is endangered, and without a healthy, engaged, and supported workforce, safer patient care will remain elusive.

Safety Is Personal [7]

Partnering with Patients and Families for the Safest Care

Workshop Leaders: Susan Edgman-Levitan and James Conway

Receiving safe care is definitely a personal experience. The harm to patients resulting from medical errors at the most vulnerable moments of their lives is a profoundly intimate experience for everyone involved. Clinicians and staff are also deeply affected when they are involved in an adverse event and frequently suffer shame, guilt, fear, and long-lasting depression.

But ensuring safety can also be shared and rewarding. The insights and perspectives of both those who experience care at its best and those who experience it at its worst can help health-care leaders, clinicians, and staff at every level make the improvements needed to create a safer and more patient-centered system.

Engaging patients and families in improving health-care safety means creating effective partnerships between those who provide care and those who receive it—at every level, including individual clinical encounters, safety committees, executive suites, boardrooms, research teams, and national policy-setting bodies. Increasing engagement through effective partnerships can yield many benefits, both in the form of improved health and outcomes for individuals and in safer and more productive work environments for health-care professionals.

Patients, families, and their advocates increasingly understand the wisdom of this partnership. Too often, standing in the way is the health-care system itself—whether by intention or not—because of its fragmentation, paternalistic professional culture, abundance of poor process design, and lack of experience on the part of health-care leaders and clinicians with practical methods of engaging patients in the safety enterprise.

While patients and families can play a critical role in preventing medical errors and reducing harm, the responsibility for safe care lies primarily with the leaders of health-care organizations and the clinicians and staff who deliver care. Many of the barriers to engagement faced by patients and families—such as lack of access to their health records, intimidation, fear of retribution, and lack of easy-to-understand tools and checklists for enhancing safe care—can only be overcome if leaders and clinicians support patients and families to become more confident and effective in their interactions with health-care providers. Many of the tools necessary to do this already exist, but the system must also provide the education and training needed by professionals and patients alike to become more effective partners.

Summary of Recommendations (Table 22.4)

Progress

With the increasing use of decision aids, patient portals, OpenNotes, care engagement plans, and the spread of Patient and Family Advisory Councils (PFACs), health-care leaders and clinicians are beginning to understand the power of engaging patients and families as integral partners. The OpenNotes program has demonstrated that patients can contribute to preventing or mitigating errors.

Patient experience data is being used more widely and effectively. Mandates from CMS, the National Committee for Quality Assurance (NCQA), and other payers for use and improvement of Consumer Assessment of Healthcare Providers and Systems (CAHPS) patient experience survey data are linked to improved performance and outcomes.

Health-care systems, hospitals, and ambulatory practices are also beginning to incorporate patient preferences into care design by

Table 22.4 Key recommendations from *Safety Is Personal: Partnering with Patients and Families for the Safest Care*

Target of recommendation	Recommendation
Leaders of health systems	Establish patient and family engagement as a core value by involving patients and families as equal partners in all organizational activities. Educate and train clinicians and staff to be effective partners; and partner with patient advocacy groups and community organizations to increase public awareness and engagement
Health-care clinicians and staff	Support patients and families to engage effectively in their own care by providing the information, training, and tools they need to manage their health conditions according to their expressed wishes Engage patients as equal partners in safety improvements and care design Support patients and families when things go wrong
Health-care policy makers	Involve patients in all policy-making committees and programs Develop, implement, and report safety metrics that foster accountability and transparency Engage patients in setting and implementing the research agenda
Patients and families and the public	Ask questions about their care and understand their medicines and care plans. They should also be instructed in basic safety steps: repeating back instructions and information to clinicians in their own words; bringing a friend or family member to all appointments; and understanding who is in charge of their care

including patients and their families as active participants in codesign and research studies funded by the Patient-Centered Outcomes Research Institute (PCORI). The internationally observed "What Matters to You?" Day aims to encourage meaningful conversations between patients, families, and providers.

Patient and family perspectives are valuable in many arenas, from design of the physical environment and care coordination plans to reporting safety concerns and participation in root cause analyses. Patient engagement should be authentic and take place across the continuum of care from the bedside to the boardroom to national policy committees. The newly established Patient Experience Policy Forum affiliated with the Beryl Institute is advocating for patient and family partnerships in codesign and policy making nationally.

Remaining Challenges

While some exemplary organizations are fully engaging patients in the care process, ample opportunities for improvement remain. Many organizations lack effective PFACs and have not devoted resources to train staff in shared decision-making practices or to offer evidence-based decision aids. The current fee-for-service payment system does not encourage clinicians to spend the time needed to communicate with patients nor to elicit their preferences.

Many organizations still lack process improvement skills to support integrating better communication into clinical workflows. As care shifts from inpatient to ambulatory and home care settings, patients and families are becoming more responsible for delivering their own care. However, they may not be well equipped to manage complicated medication regimens, activities of daily living, medical devices, or infection control procedures.

Overwhelming evidence indicates that collecting patient feedback and including patients as equal partners in their care support improvement in both patient experience of care and clinical outcomes. Opportunities remain to partner with patients, families, and communities to accelerate improvement in education, patient satisfaction, and quality of care.

Shining a Light [8]

Safer Health Care Through Transparency

Workshop Leaders: Gary Kaplan and Robert Wachter

During the course of health care's patient safety and quality movements, the impact of transparency—the free, uninhibited flow of information that is open to the scrutiny of others—has been far more positive than many had anticipated, and the harms of transparency have been far fewer than many had feared. Yet important obstacles to transparency remain, ranging from concerns that individuals and organizations will be treated unfairly after being transparent to more practical matters related to identifying appropriate measures on which to be transparent and creating an infrastructure for reporting and disseminating the lessons learned from others' data.

To address the issue of transparency in the context of patient safety, the National Patient Safety Foundation's Lucian Leape Institute held two roundtable discussions involving a wide variety of stakeholders representing myriad perspectives. In the discussions and in this report, the choice was made to focus on four domains of transparency:

- Transparency between clinicians and patients (illustrated by disclosure after medical errors)
- Transparency among clinicians themselves (illustrated by peer review and other mechanisms to share information within health-care delivery organizations)
- Transparency of health-care organizations with one another (illustrated by regional or national collaboratives)
- Transparency of both clinicians and organizations with the public (illustrated by public reporting of quality and safety data)

One key insight was the degree to which these four domains are interrelated. For example, creating environments in which clinicians are open and honest with each other about their errors within organizations (which can lead to important system changes to prevent future errors) can be thwarted if these clinicians believe they will be treated unfairly should the same errors be publicly disclosed. These tensions cannot be wished away; instead, they must be forthrightly addressed by institutional and policy leaders.

In this report, the NPSF Lucian Leape Institute comes down strongly on the side of transparency in all four domains. The consensus of the roundtable discussants and the Institute is that the evidence supports the premise that greater transparency throughout the system is not only ethically correct but will lead to improved outcomes, fewer errors, more satisfied patients, and lower costs. The mechanisms for these improvements are several and include the ability of transparency to support accountability, stimulate improvements in quality and safety, promote trust and ethical behavior, and facilitate patient choice.

In the report, more than three dozen specific recommendations are offered to individual clinicians, leaders of health-care delivery organizations (e.g., CEOs, board members), and policy makers.

If transparency were a medication, it would be a blockbuster, with billions of dollars in sales and accolades the world over. While it is crucial to be mindful of the obstacles to transparency and the tensions—and the fact that many stakeholders benefit from our current largely nontransparent system—our review convinces us that a health-care system that embraces transparency across the four domains will be one that produces safer care, better outcomes, and more trust among all of the involved parties. Notwithstanding the potential rewards, making this happen will depend on powerful, courageous leadership and an underlying culture of safety.

Summary of Recommendations (Table 22.5)

Progress

Today, the call for greater transparency in health care is growing louder. Consumers have begun to post reviews of their physicians, care teams, and health-care organizations on online review platforms. Moreover, some health-care systems are now collecting and posting information from patient experience surveys at the service or physician level. Recently, several health systems have begun to provide forums for free-response comments online, often with positive results.

The 2005 Patient Safety and Quality Improvement Act and the rise of patient safety organizations (PSOs) have facilitated increased transparency among clinicians and health-care organizations. Additionally, collaboratives like Solutions for Patient Safety (SPS), a network of more than 130 children's hospitals working together to eliminate serious harm, have shown compelling evidence that sharing data, successes, and failures can markedly accelerate learning and improvement.

Health care is also seeing greater transparency between patients and clinicians in the aftermath of adverse events. A growing number of communication and resolution programs have been established, fueled by growing evidence that prompt disclosure, honesty, and

Table 22.5 Key recommendations from *Shining a Light: Safer Health Care Through Transparency*

Target of recommendation	Recommendation
All stakeholders	Ensure disclosure of conflicts of interest, and provide patients with reliable information in a form that is useful to them
	Create organizational cultures that support transparency, shared learning, and core competencies regarding communication with patients and families, other clinicians, and the public
Leaders and boards	Prioritize transparency and safety, and frequently review comprehensive safety performance data
	Link hiring, firing, promotion, and compensation to results in cultural transformation and transparency
Governmental agencies	Develop data sources for collection of safety data, improve standards and training materials for core competencies, and develop an all-payer database and robust medical device registries
Clinicians	Inform patients of clinician's experience, conflicts of interest, and role in care, and provide patients with a full description of all the alternatives for tests and treatments and the pros and cons for each
	Provide patients with full information about all planned tests and treatments
Hospitals and health systems	Provide patients with full access to their medical records, and include patients and family members in interdisciplinary bedside rounds
Hospitals and health systems, health professionals	Provide patients and families with full information about any harm resulting from treatment, followed by apology and fair resolution
	Provide patients and clinicians support when they are involved in an incident. Include patients/family members in event reporting and in root cause analysis
Hospital and health leaders	Create a safe, supportive culture for caregivers to be transparent and accountable to each other
	Create multidisciplinary processes and forms for reporting, analyzing, and sharing data
	Create processes to hold individuals accountable for risky or disruptive behavior
Health-care organizations, hospital associations, PSOs	Have clear mechanisms for sharing and adopting best practices, for example, by participating in state and regional collaboratives
Hospitals and health-care organizations	Report and publicly display measures used to monitor quality and safety, and clearly communicate to the public about performance

apology following patient injury can decrease medical malpractice liability and improve the satisfaction of all parties. Toolkits are now available to promote such programs.

Remaining Challenges

Many challenges to achieving full transparency remain. A recent survey found that less than 40% of quality and safety leaders rated their board's understanding of disclosure and apology as "high," and even fewer felt their boards had a comprehensive understanding of safety concepts related to transparency about error and harm. Transparency within organizations and between providers requires creating an environment of trust as well as improving technology and processes to ensure they are efficient and effective and promote regular open and honest communication and data sharing.

Transparency with the public is equally challenging. Hospital and clinician concerns about litigation; reputational costs; and the accuracy, interpretability, and comprehensiveness of safety metrics need to be addressed. Additionally, national rating systems and websites, including Leapfrog and U.S. News & World Report, share few common scores and often generate more confusion than clarity. For example, as of 2015 no hospital was rated as a high performer by all four major national US rating systems. In the future, data must be understandable and actionable for both patients and provider organizations.

As more organizations publicly share their quality, safety, and patient experience data, transparency will be increasingly demanded by all stakeholders. To benefit patients as well as care providers, organizations will need to prepare their boards, clinicians, and staff for a more transparent health-care system. Transparency at these levels will eventually facilitate decision-making about where to receive care and where to work, but a long road lies ahead to make this comparable and uniform across all health entities.

The last of the five white papers was published in 2015. Printed copies of all of them were circulated widely to CEOs and patient safety leaders of schools and health-care organizations, patient safety specialists, and members of the roundtables, who you will recall included individuals and leaders of organizations that could implement the recommendations.

While all of the reports were well-received, it is impossible to know their impact. Implementing the recommendations requires strong leadership and major cultural changes. Stimulating those changes, of course, is what we were trying to do with the white papers by providing the evidence, the arguments, and the tools for change. Some minds were undoubtedly changed. The foundation was laid for the transformations needed to make health care safe.

Transforming Health Care: A Compendium

While the white papers got good reviews and wide circulation, we were well aware that their lengths would be barriers to reading them for many who would benefit from them. So, when the last of the five white papers was finished in 2015, we wrote a compendium that brought together the executive summary and recommendations for each of the five topics, plus additional recommendations for getting started on making the changes: *Transforming Health Care: A Compendium of Reports from the National Patient Safety Foundation's Lucian Leape Institute* [2].

Our hope was that this 30-page document would not only make some of the many lessons and critical insights we had gathered more accessible, but that it would also stimulate readers to read the original monographs. Like the white papers, *Transforming Health Care: A Compendium* is available free on the IHI website.

Members

Since its inception, the membership of the Institute has changed as new members were added and others retired. Early on, we invited patient advocate *Susan Edgman-Levitan*, Executive Director of the John D. Stoeckle Center for Primary Care Innovation at the MGH to join us. To bring in outside perspectives, we were fortunate to attract *Paul O'Neill*, former CEO of Alcoa and 72nd United States Secretary of the Treasury, and *James Guest*, head of Consumers Union. *Janet Corrigan*, former IOM staff director for *To Err is Human* joined us shortly thereafter, as did *Robert M. Wachter*, founder of the hospitalist specialty and Associate Chair Department of Medicine, UCSF, and *Charles Vincent*, UK leader of patient safety research of the University of Oxford.

Later additions included *Amy Edmondson*, Professor at Harvard Business School; *Sue Sheridan*, Director of Patient Engagement, Patient-Centered Outcomes Research Institute; *David Michaels*, former Head of the Occupational Safety and Health Administration; *Gregg Meyer*, Chief Clinical Officer Of Mass General Brigham; and *Joanne Disch*, former Chair of the Board of Advocate-Aurora Health System.

In 2014, *Tejal Gandhi* became president of the Institute when Diane Pinakiewicz retired. *Gary Kaplan*, CEO of Virginia Mason Medical Center, joined LLI when he stepped down as chair of the Board of NPSF. He took over as chair of the Institute when I retired in 2015.

In addition to the five white papers, LLI pursued a number of other strategic efforts to motivate change for patient safety. From the beginning, the annual fund-raising gala had a major educational component. Prior to the evening social event, we presented a full afternoon symposium that provided a variety of unique learning opportunities for attendees, such as an open forum where they could hear presentations and question LLI members and breakout sessions on specific patient safety topics. The evening program featured an address by a world-renowned safety expert.

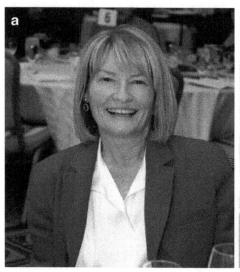
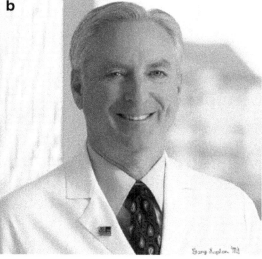

(**a**) Susan Edgman-Levitan and (**b**) Gary Kaplan.

The Institute held a fund-raising gala each year, which included an afternoon educational program conducted by the members and an evening banquet with a featured celebrity speaker. These were highly successful events attracting several hundred attendees each year.

LLI members also participated as faculty in the leadership course and other activities at the annual NPSF Congress. A highly popular feature was the annual LLI panel where several members discussed a current patient safety topic.

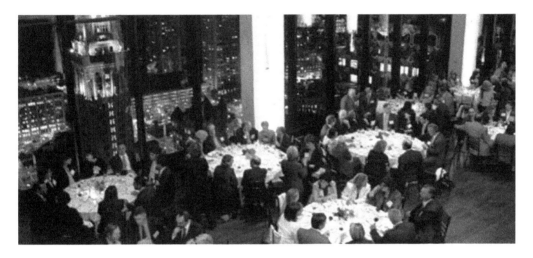

LLI Gala. Source: National Patient Safety Foundation (now Institute for Healthcare Improvement).

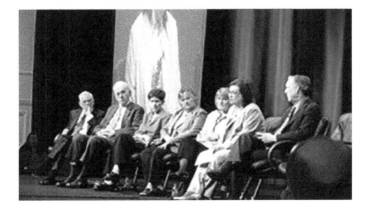

LLI Panel. From left to right: Paul O'Neill, Jim Conway, Carolyn Clancy, Pam Thompson, Susan Edgman-Levitan, Julie Morath, Gary Kaplan. (Source: National Patient Safety Foundation (now Institute for Healthcare Improvement).

Later Work

The "Must Do" List

As the concept of responding to errors by treating them as systems problems instead of blaming individuals became widely accepted, some applied the idea to all failures, and the term "no-blame" culture emerged. This misconception was countered by the definition and promotion of the "Just Culture" as defined by Reason and David Marx, who distinguished error from negligence, reckless behavior, and intentional rule violations [9, 10].

Rule violations can be tricky, since there are times when a non-standard response is required in an individual situation. These should be dealt with on an individual basis. But most violations are not in that category; they result from individual preferences, inconvenience, or resistance to change. A fair and just culture demands that such individual violators be held accountable. Unfortunately, health-care organizations varied widely in which practices they placed in this category and how they responded to violations. Few consistently enforced meaningful sanctions.

Members of LLI were of a single mind that certain safe practices were of such undisputed value that they should be universally followed and that sanctions should be applied to violators, i.e., some failures are truly "blameworthy." The practices in this category are those that (1) are *effective* at preventing an important harm, (2) have substantial *impact*, (3) are *feasible* to comply with and audit, and (4) have been accepted as a *standard* by the NQF and professional consensus. These are safety practices that have sufficiently compelling supportive evidence that clinicians should not have the right of an individual veto. We called them "Must Do" practices.

These concepts were laid out by Bob Wachter in a paper on the Health Affairs Blog, *The 'Must Do' List: Certain Patient Safety Rules Should Not Be Elective*, that provided the rationale for this approach. It identified two practices that currently met the criteria: hand hygiene and influenza vaccination for health-care workers [11].

We called on health-care organizations to expect 100 percent adherence to these practices, to sanction violators, and to be willing to terminate clinicians for deliberate and repeated noncompliance with either of these practices. We recommended that expectation of universal compliance with required practices be included in bylaws and clinician compacts. We also called on the Joint Commission and CMS and other regulators and accreditors to adopt these standards.

Financial Costs of Patient Safety

One of the arguments given by health-care organizations for not moving ahead more aggressively to improve patient safety was that they could not afford it, that implementing new practices costs more than they save. As measurement of adverse events began to take hold, however, research showed that the costs of the additional care and prolonged hospital stays caused by preventable injuries are substantial. The additional cost has been estimated at $16–18 billion annually [12] but is probably considerably higher because of underreporting. The cost of hospital-acquired infections alone has been estimated as more than $10 billion a year [13].

Hospitals were able to absorb these costs because they could bill for additional days and services caused by the injury. That began to change during the Obama Administration with the move toward value-based purchasing. Under bundled and capitated payment programs, the marginal costs of treating injuries are not compensated, eroding hospital margins. Suddenly reducing those harms became more attractive.

LLI decided to write a paper to encourage purchasers to promote safety through financial incentives and identify what further steps could be taken to strengthen marketplace incentives. In *On the safe side: the move to value-based payment models could mean improvements in patient safety*, Corrigan et al. pointed the way [14]. In addition to the direct benefit to patients from reducing adverse events, creating a safe environment enhances workplace productivity, morale, and retention. In the competitive marketplace, improved safety enhances the system's reputation and ability to increase market share. Malpractice costs will decline.

We called on executives to increase awareness of the costs by including estimates of the direct and indirect expenses associated with medical errors in financial statements shared with trustees, leadership, staff, and the public and to ensure that a portion of their organizations' capital budgets are allocated for investments in safety such as barcoding. When the financial consequences of unsafe care are accounted for, it is clear that investing in patient safety is both the right thing to do and the profitable thing to do.

Collaboration with American College of Healthcare Executives

As health-care organizations gained experience with changing systems, it became increasingly clear that more extensive culture changes were needed, and this required strong leadership. LLI began to look for strategies to engage and motivate health-care systems leaders.

In 2015, LLI approached the American College of Healthcare Executives (ACHE) regarding a joint effort. The timing was fortuitous. Under new leadership, ACHE was seeking to establish itself as a thought leader in the executive space. We formed a partnership to sponsor two roundtables on leading a culture of safety, co-chaired by leaders of the two organizations.

The participants in these roundtables, held in 2016, included CEOs and patient safety officers from a number of hospitals and systems, large and small, academics, and leaders of professional organizations, such as the AONE, AHA, ANA, and IHI, and leadership consulting organizations.

The work of the roundtables was summarized with recommendations in *Leading a Culture of Safety: A Blueprint for Success*, published jointly by ACHE and LLI [15]. This is probably the most comprehensive and useful guide for creating a culture of safety. It is described in more detail in the next chapter.

Since 2015, the end of the period of this history, NPSF merged with IHI, which committed to continuing support of LLI. Major LLI initiatives since then include:

- Partnering with NORC at the University of Chicago to conduct a survey of American's experience with medical errors and views on patient safety [16].
- *Transforming concepts in patient safety*: a report on progress in each of the five areas since they were formulated in 2009 [3].
- Framework for Effective Board Governance of Health System Quality [17].
- The Salzburg Statement on Moving Measurement into Action: Global Principles for Measuring Patient Safety [18].

Conclusion

How much impact the white papers and other LLI initiatives have had on making health care safer is impossible to know. The roundtables for the five transforming concepts and the one engaging leaders with ACHE were highly motivating for the participants. These key organizational and policy leaders—the "movers and shakers"—were enthusiastic participants, and the discussions clearly advanced thinking about each of the issues in practical and actionable ways.

The roundtables and white papers also appear to have significantly increased awareness of the complex issues in patient safety and deepened understanding of these issues for many other leaders in health care. They truly changed the conversation and helped put patient safety on everyone's agenda. To that extent, the Institute has made great progress in meeting its charge, to "define strategic paths and calls to action for the field of patient safety."

References

1. Leape L, Berwick D, Clancy C, et al. Transforming healthcare: a safety imperative. Qual Saf Health Care. 2009;18(6):424–8.
2. National Patient Safety Foundation's Lucian Leape Institute. Transforming health care: a compendium of reports from the NPSF Lucian Leape Institute. Boston: National Patient Safety Foundation; 2016.
3. Gandhi TK, Kaplan GS, Leape L, et al. Transforming concepts in patient safety: a progress report. BMJ Qual Saf. 2018;27(12):1019–26.
4. National Patient Safety Foundation. Unmet needs: teaching physicians to provide safe patient care. Boston; 2010.
5. Lucian Leape Institute. Order from Chaos: accelerating care integration. Boston: National Patient Safety Foundation; 2012.
6. Lucian Leape Institute. Through the eyes of the workforce: creating joy, meaning, and safer health care. Boston: National Patient Safety Foundation; 2013.
7. National Patient Safety Foundation's Lucian Leape Institute. Safety is personal: partnering with patients and families for the safest care. Boston: National Patient Safety Foundation; 2014.
8. National Patient Safety Foundation's Lucian Leape Institute. Shining a light: safer health care through transparency. Boston: National Patient Safety Foundation; 2015.
9. Reason JT. Managing the risks of organizational accidents. Aldershot, Hants; Brookfield: Ashgate; 1997.
10. Marx D. Patient safety and the "just culture": a primer for health care executives. New York. 17 Apr 17, 2001.

11. Wachter RM. The 'Must Do' list: certain patient safety rules should not be elective. In. *Health Affairs Blog.* Vol 2020: Health Affairs; 20 Aug 2015.

12. U.S. Department of Health and Human Services. New HHS data shows major strides made in patient safety, leading to improved care and savings. 7 May 2014.

13. Zimlichman E, Henderson D, Tamir O, et al. Health care-associated infections: a meta-analysis of costs and financial impact on the US health care system. JAMA Intern Med. 2013;173(22):2039–46.

14. Corrigan JM, Wakeam E, Gandhi TK, Leape LL. On the safe side: the move to value-based payment models could mean improvements in patient safety. Healthc Financ Manage. 2015;69(8):94.

15. American College of Healthcare Executives and IHI/NPSF Lucian Leape Institute. Leading a culture of safety: a blueprint for success. Boston: American College of Healthcare Executives and Institute for Healthcare Improvement; 2017.

16. NORC at the University of Chicago and IHI/NPSF Lucian Leape Institute. Americans' experiences with medical errors and views on patient safety. Cambridge: Institute for Healthcare Improvement and NORC at the University of Chicago; 2017.

17. Daley Ullem E, Gandhi TK, Mate K, Whittington J, Renton M, Huebner J. Framework for Effective Board Governance of Health System Quality. IHI White Paper. Boston: Institute for Healthcare Improvement; 2018.

18. Salzburg Global Seminar & Institute for Healthcare Improvement. The Salzburg statement on moving measurement into action: global principles for measuring patient safety: Institute for Healthcare Improvement and Salzburg Global Seminar; 2019.

23

What is a Culture of Safety and How to Build it?

In 2020, the coronavirus pandemic killed 1,800,000 people, 346,000 of them Americans. In that same year, if recent estimates are correct, about the same number died as a result of medical errors, all despite the enormous effort of the past 20 years to eliminate preventable harm, an effort that has involved people at all levels: policy makers, government agencies, oversight bodies, quality improvement organizations, major health-care systems, and thousands of providers and caregivers on the frontline.

Many injuries have been prevented, and thousands of lives have been saved. Fewer people suffer from hospital-acquired infections and medication errors, surgical complications, and falls in the hospital. But the overall number of preventable injuries has hardly budged. The relentless advances in medical science and the constantly changing demands of the environments in which we deliver care create new opportunities for harm faster than we can keep up.

We have learned a great deal. Driven by the concept that the cause of errors and unintended harm is not bad people, but bad systems, we have been engaged in an immense experiment testing myriad ways to make those systems changes. It has truly been a paradigm shift. Early efforts focused on changing processes at the level of the care unit or hospital. These were initially ad hoc responses to local problems, but with time an impressive repertoire has been developed of standardized practices of proven effectiveness that can be widely adopted (see Chap. 11).

Several large systems, such as the Veterans Health Administration, Ascension, Kaiser-Permanente, and others, expanded the use of these proven practices to all of their hospitals and clinics. Collaboratives have been developed that brought together quality improvement teams from a region or nationally to work together to implement a practice. Some of these were spectacularly successful, virtually eliminating a major threat in those hospitals [1].

Despite these impressive successes, the painful fact is that with few exceptions (such as two-factor identification of patients, barcoding of medications, and perhaps hand hygiene), most of this awesome array of standardized effective practices has not been adopted by the majority of providers and health-care organizations. Health care is still stunningly unsafe.

But even if the adoption problem could be solved, relying on universal implementation of specific practices is not likely to be an effective strategy for achieving safe health care. The potential number required must be in the thousands, and the complexities of health care ensure that new hazards will constantly arise for which there are no known practices.

If the experience of other industries that have succeeded in becoming safe is a guide, it will require much more than changing our practices to prevent specific harms. It will require changing our culture. A change that was called for in the earliest writings on patient safety [2] and in the legendary IOM report [3].

What are we talking about? What is culture, and what is the culture change that is required?

What Is Culture?

The word culture has been used, abused, and misused a great deal in the health-care literature. A major disagreement, especially in the UK, centers on whether the culture of a group should be defined in terms of its attitudes, assumptions, values, and beliefs or in terms of its actions, "how we do things around here." Is culture who we *are* or what we *do*? I believe the evidence is clear that it is both – and that each determines the other, which is the point of this chapter.

For example, from time immemorial, a well-established espoused value and assumption about physician behavior was that the physician had the sole authority to make treatment decisions, irrespective of external guidelines or internal contrary advice. The result – the practice – was deference to their authority. When that practice has been changed, when a hospital adopts adherence to standards as a condition of practice, not only does the "way we do things" change, so do, gradually, the attitudes and the values of the culture overall.

In anthropology, culture refers to social behavior in different societies or the knowledge, beliefs, and customs of their members expressed in their traditions, mythology, or religion. Nation-states pride themselves on their cultures, their traditions, their "solidarity" (or lack of it), and their particular religious commitment. We also speak of culture as a term of human refinement to differentiate elite from others.

Within societies we speak of the culture of subgroups, such as the military, medicine, "hippies," or the culture of a firm such as IBM or Apple. We note regional cultures such as those of the South or Midwest. In all these contexts, culture reflects the deep shared values and assumptions that guide us in what we should and should not do. Those values are expressed in behavior, "how we do things around here."

When we think of "how we do things around here" in health care, the focus is not just on patient care and the provider-patient interface but also includes the relationships and interactions of all who work in the care delivery setting. Individual medical specialties, nursing, pharmacy, etc. have strong subcultures, but it is predominantly the *organizational culture* of the hospital or clinic that determines how patients are cared for.

Most of what we know about organizational culture comes from studies of other industries. The work of Edgar Schein is preeminent [4]. Schein notes that three elements define an organization's culture: its shared *assumptions*; its *espoused values*, i.e., what a group ideally wants to be and wishes to present itself to the public; and the day-to-day *behaviors*. Culture includes everything we do in an organization; it makes sense of what we do, it provides stability.

The shared assumptions run deep. They are the "truth" as perceived by the organization's members: their beliefs about human nature, such as whether people are intrinsically self-motivated or motivated by money, their perceptions of reality, and their concept of mission. In health care, shared assumptions include a commitment to responding to emergencies and putting the patient's interest first. They are the unwritten rules.

Espoused values include such things as individualism, respect for authority, and working hard. Behaviors are the visible manifestations of the culture, the rituals and how we treat one another, labelled by Schein as "artifacts" [4]. Others have used the term *safety climate* to refer to these expressions of the culture.

Schein summarizes this in a definition of culture that is widely accepted as capturing the essential aspects: "A pattern of shared basic assumptions that was learned by a group as it solved its problems of external adaptation and internal integration, that has worked well enough to be considered valid and, therefore, to be taught to new members as the correct way to perceive, think, and feel in relation to those problems" [4].

In large organizations such as hospitals, the individual units, services, and divisions also have their own cultures. These subcultures share some of the organization's values and assumptions, but not necessarily all, with the result that members of one unit may engage in behaviors that differ substantially from those in another. For example, when a nurse makes an error, whether the unit's nursing culture is supportive or blaming affects whether they will report the error so it becomes known and can be investigated. The culture in the ICU may be very different from that in the emergency room or from another ICU down the hall.

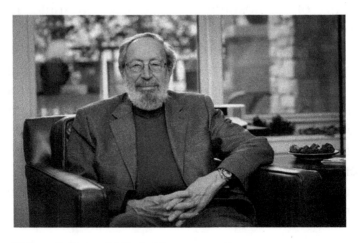

Edgar Schein. (All rights reserved)

A Culture of Safety

What is a *culture of safety*? The term was first used by the International Nuclear Safety Advisory Group report following the 1986 disaster at the Chernobyl Nuclear Power Plant, the cause of which was attributed to a breakdown in the organization's safety culture [5, 6].

A useful definition was later put forth by the UK Health and Safety Commission:

> The safety culture of an organization is the product of the individual and group values, attitudes, competencies and patterns of behavior that determine the commitment to, and the style and proficiency of, an organization's health and safety programs. Organizations with a positive safety culture are characterized by communications founded on mutual trust, by shared perceptions of the importance of safety, and by confidence in the efficacy of preventive measures [7].

One of the earliest and most respected students of organizational culture, James Reason, of the University of Manchester, UK, identified five components that characterize a culture of safety [8]. It must be:

- An *informed culture*: It needs data about incidents and near misses.
- A *reporting culture*: Workers must feel it is safe to report and that it makes a difference.
- A *just culture*: People are rewarded for providing essential safety information, but deliberate breaking of the rules is not tolerated.
- A *flexible culture*: The organization can reconfigure itself in response to a new danger, such as moving from hierarchical structure to a flattened structure as needed.
- A *learning culture*: It is able to draw the right conclusions from its information system and has the will to implement major reforms when needed.

One follows from another. An informed culture can only be built on the foundations of a reporting culture. This, in turn, depends upon establishing a just culture. Flexibility and learning are only possible if the other components are established. But none of this is possible without openness and trust.

As Schein points out, a culture of safety can only exist within the broader culture of a health-care organization that is committed to providing patients with the experience of high-quality effective care, delivered efficiently by valued and engaged workers. While in other industries the safety focus is on *workers*, in health care it is primarily on the patient, but to succeed it must also include worker safety.

Characteristics of a Safe Culture

Unfortunately, few health-care organizations have seriously striven to become a safe culture. What should it look like? What are the characteristics of a safe culture in health care?

At the *organizational* level, in a culture of safety everyone shares a commitment to the goal of zero harm and to the continuing improvement and innovation that are required to get there – to the belief that anything is possible. There is a sense of individual responsibility at every level, that safety is everyone's job. Leaders exemplify these commitments and motivate others to share them. Their sincerity of purpose, consistency, and transparency inspire trust.

The individual is valued, and every voice is heard. Leaders seek to follow the advice of Paul O'Neill, the highly successful CEO of Alcoa, who taught that every worker, every day, should come to work feeling they are respected regardless of rank or expertise, supported to do their work well, and appreciated for what they contribute.

At the *operational* level, in a culture of safety people work in teams and are open and trusting of one another. They share the mission of providing care that is free of harm. There is a commitment to standard work, i.e., finding the best way to do something and everyone doing it, yet they are open to changing it to make it better. Innovation and improvement are part of everyday work and are everyone's responsibility. They give meaning to work. Patients are fully engaged as partners in their care and in improvement.

At the *individual* level, in a safe culture, workers feel valued and supported. Their deep sense of individual responsibility for safety is expressed not only by being careful but by being alert and looking for hazards, "accidents waiting to happen." Errors, harms, near misses, and hazards are promptly reported because they know they will be taken seriously, promptly investigated, and acted upon.

A culture of safety is a *learning culture*. It is an environment where everyone is aware of how far their work falls short of what it could be and is committed to improve. A learning culture is characterized by its members' ability to self-reflect and identify strengths and defects [9]. People pay attention, notice problems, and reflect on them. Problems are analyzed, and solutions are imagined and created. Changes are implemented.

Schein emphasizes that a learning culture is based on positive assumptions about human nature: that human nature is good and that people will learn if it is psychologically safe to do so. There is commitment to learning to learn, to truth as discovered by inquiry, to full and open communication, to systems thinking [4]. A learning culture is based on trust, transparency, and reliability.

A Just Culture

A culture of safety is also a *fair and just culture*. What does this mean? From the beginning, the fundamental aim of the patient safety movement has been to shift the focus from the individual to the system when things go wrong. Some (not your author) have referred to this as a "no-blame" approach. For the vast majority of iatrogenic harms, probably 90% or more, this is appropriate. The harm was unintentional and resulted from poor system design. The caregiver is truly the "second victim."

But some errors and some injuries are caused by intentional acts. For these a no-blame approach is inappropriate.

If the individual intended to cause harm, the act is assault and should be dealt with by the legal system. Fortunately, assault is exceedingly rare in health care (serial murders, etc.). The much more common intentional act is *rule breaking* in which the caregiver does not intend harm, but deliberately fails to follow a standard procedure.

This form of violation is actually quite common. Because of time and workload pressures, nurses and doctors often "cut corners" to get their patients taken care of, especially if the rule doesn't make sense, doesn't seem to apply in this case, or prevents them from getting their work done. But even if the act seemed justified, the caregiver will feel ashamed if it harms the patient because they will realize they have "done something wrong."

These cases should be carefully investigated. If the broken rule is a bad rule, or unworkable, it should be changed, by a process that involves all stakeholders. If the existing rule is good and necessary, education may be necessary; if time pressures or workloads are the issue, these should be addressed. On the other hand, if a violation results just from the caregiver's personal preference or convenience, discipline may be indicated, especially if there is a pattern of such behavior.

Seeing that indefensible repeated violations have consequences is important for co-workers in two ways. They see that justice is done – the person didn't "get away with it" – and it reinforces their own rule-abiding behavior. A just culture is the necessary balance to a systems approach [8, 10].

The term safety culture is sometimes confused with safety *climate*, which is its outward manifestation – its visible evidence, or "artifacts" as Schein puts it. Safety climate more appropriately refers to the *perception* of the culture, what people think about themselves and "what we do around here." It is what we measure when we attempt to measure safety culture [11].

High-Reliability Organizations

Much has been written about *high-reliability organizations* (*HRO*) and whether they are the model for a safe culture. The concept is based on a series of studies in the early 1990s by Roberts and colleagues of highly hazardous industries, such as aviation and nuclear power, that had succeeded in becoming extremely safe [12]. While it is true that, unlike health care, these industries had strong business cases for safety – they would be out of business if unsafe – the fact is that they are amazingly successful.

Weick and Sutcliffe identified five characteristics that account for the success of HRO, which they label *collective mindfulness*: (1) preoccupation with failure, the continual looking for and reporting of hazards; (2) reluctance to simplify, not accepting the obvious explanation for a failure; (3) sensitivity to operations, paying attention to issues at the frontline; (4) commitment to resilience, the ability to detect errors, react, and recover; and (5) deference to expertise, the flattening of the hierarchy in an emergency so that the most qualified person is in charge, regardless of seniority [13].

Collective mindfulness leads to the essential behavior for safety, which is that everyone understands that even small failures can lead to catastrophic outcomes and accepts responsibility both for identifying hazards early and for correcting them before harm occurs [13].

In other industries, HROs have achieved a culture of safety and enviable outcomes. The idea of applying these principles to health care is attractive [14]. Certainly these characteristics of structure, attitude, and expertise need to be part of the changes in quality of care and experience that make health care safe.

The originator of the concept of HROs, Karlene Roberts, also attributes much of their success to the emphasis on *relational* aspects of the culture: interpersonal responsibility, person-centeredness, being supportive of co-workers, friendliness, openness in personal relations, creativity, credibility, interpersonal trust, and resiliency [12, 15].

The Problem

Most health-care organizations fall woefully short of achieving a culture of safety. With just a few exceptions, hospitals and health-care systems, including some of the most highly regarded academic health centers, have settled for implementing some safe practices; the culture is unchanged.

In a safe culture, there is a strong commitment to the goal of zero harm and to the continuing improvement and innovation that is required to get there. In health care, safety is too often an afterthought or at best a distant second fiddle to the bottom line. There is no sense of commitment, no goal of zero harm. Deliberate unsafe care is often tolerated, especially among big earners.

In a safe culture, safety information systems collect data on incidents and near misses. Reporting of adverse events or hazards is encouraged and leads to investigation, analysis, and, where possible, redesign of a process or system to eliminate the risk. In health care, many institutions have established reporting system and a process for root cause analysis of events to meet accreditation requirements, but their use is often perfunctory. Now 25 years after hospitals were urged to stop blaming people for errors, nearly half of nurses surveyed by the Joint Commission say they do not report errors because of fear that they or a colleague will be punished.

In a safe culture, workers feel valued, supported, and empowered. They have a sense of ownership, of responsibility, to prevent harm and work well in teams. Sadly, in health care this sense of responsibility and empowerment has long been inhibited by a hierarchical system that devalues their contributions and makes working in teams difficult. It is a culture of low expectations and low accountability.

Why Changing Culture Is so Hard to Do

Creating a safe culture is the key part of the transformation that a health-care organization must undergo overall to reliably provide a patient experience of high-quality, effective, and efficient care. Under the best of circumstances, these are difficult changes to carry off, but health care also offers a staggering array of barriers to change.

The first has been *resistance* by the key members of the workforce: physicians. Products of an educational system that traditionally emphasized personal responsibility for patient care, many viewed standardization as a threat to their independence and personal judgment. Giving up control and sharing responsibility by working in teams were hard to do.

Fortunately, that has begun to change. Younger physicians have learned the importance of quality improvement and are amenable to working in teams. They "get it" and now constitute a significant majority of physicians.

The second major barrier to change is an incredibly complicated demand/incentive *payment system* that compels hospitals – i.e., doctors and nurses – to document that they meet quality and volume requirements. The result is an extensive, and, for caregivers, depressing, set of demands on their time that compete directly with their primary mission of taking care of patients.

This oppressive payment system is the product of two forces that changed dramatically in the past several decades: the ability to measure safety and quality and the rising cost of care.

Twenty years ago, as the quality and safety movement was gaining steam, many complained about the paucity of good measures. For safety, what were the errors and systems failures we should focus on? For quality, the IOM called for care that was safe, efficient, timely, patient-centered, efficient, and equitable [16]. But, again, how would we know? Well, in the past 20 years we've developed methods for measuring all of these. More are needed, but thanks to an impressive effort by quality and safety researchers we can now measure quite a bit.

The other major driver of demand/incentive payment changes is *costs*, which have risen dramatically since the middle of the twentieth century primarily as the result of awesome improvements in diagnosis and treatment that have been heavily weighted toward expensive technologies. Magnetic resonance imaging, PET scans, and surgical robots, for example, cost health care millions of dollars a year. A new "miracle" drug may cost hundreds of thousands of dollars a year for a single patient.

Facing the need to contain costs, payers and regulators seized on available measures to assess performance and used them for accreditation and for value-based financial incentives. Lowered reimbursement rates force physicians to see more patients (production pressure).

A particularly painful example for physicians resulted from the generous incentives provided by the government for adoption of the electronic health record (EHR). When computerized records were being developed, many of us were enthusiastic about their potential to improve the quality of care, such as by reducing medication errors and making standardized clinical information available. A number of private companies rose to the opportunity, each with its own product, most of them built around systems they already had for billing and financial management. Not only were these clumsy, inefficient, and non-user-friendly, they were proprietary and thus would not communicate with one another.

Finally, the government stepped in—not to regulate and standardize systems as many of us had hoped, but to promote their use through a massive subsidy for the implementation of these mostly proprietary systems by hospitals and physicians. Because most of these EHRs are poorly designed, the result has been a huge increase in the time that physicians must spend in documentation.

The resulting burdens of using the EHR, increased production pressure, and loss of control are widely considered to be major factors in the dissatisfaction and burnout that has become increasingly common among health workers. We have created an environment where many nurses, doctors, and allied health staff are too exhausted, too disillusioned, and too burned out to have the interest or the energy to engage in efforts to change. There is little time for reflection, improvement, or preventing errors.

In addition to physician resistance and perverse payment incentives, a third barrier to creating a culture of safety stems from *financial threats to institutional survival*. In our predominantly fee-for-service system, economic survival of a hospital depends on the number of services provided and how much they are paid for them. To control costs, government payments—Medicare and Medicaid—are below market for virtually all services. Commercial insurance companies pay much better—sometimes multiples of Medicare reimbursement. They also negotiate rates with hospitals.

In this system, large hospitals increase their income by attracting more patients through providing ever more sophisticated and expensive treatments. Although they have many Medicare patients, large hospitals receive the major share of their income from commercial insurers with whom they negotiate rates.

Smaller hospitals lose on both counts. They are unable to attract more patients with increased services, and they lack the clout to negotiate higher rates with insurance companies. Safety net hospitals, formerly city hospitals for the indigent, and rural hospitals fare even worse. They depend almost totally on local government support and Medicaid, both at "bare-bones" levels.

In all hospitals, the CEO is under constant financial pressure—beholden to "the bottom line." The large expensive hospitals, like other corporations, vie for increased market share by providing additional services. If they become the dominant provider in a region, they can exercise monopoly power and can raise their prices. While technically "not for profit," they generate large profits, which they use to expand their services and to increase the pay of their physicians and, especially, their CEOs. According to Forbes, in 2019 the top 13 nonprofit hospitals and systems paid their CEOS between $five million and $21.6 million; the next 61 paid CEOs between $1 and five million [17].

The fourth barrier to changing culture, compounding all the others, is the incredibly *complex nature* of health care. No other industry comes close. The client—the patient—may suffer from an almost infinite number and variety of diseases. In addition, patients also vary widely in what they bring to the therapeutic encounter in terms of genetic makeup, physical and mental health, and the effect of the living environment where they receive most of their care.

Matching the number and variety of diseases is an incredible number and variety of treatments, using modalities as varied as chemicals (drugs), electromagnetic waves, surgery, robots, and computers. Compounding this is a lack of standardization of use. Each form of treatment can be—and often is—employed according to the judgment, or whim, of the provider. The result is an almost infinite number of ways things can go wrong [18].

Finally, those who *provide* care are a diverse group. In addition to doctors, nurses, and pharmacists, many other workers, such as therapists, aides, clerical staff, and support staff, are essential personnel who make a hospital work. There are 180 specialties and subspecialties in medicine alone, each with its unique knowledge, skills, and approach to patient care.

The complexity of health care and the formidable array of regulatory and financial forces impacting it are awesome. Changing the culture will require that these interests be aligned and that public-private partnerships be developed. But what, exactly, do we want a hospital to do? We have a clear idea of what a culture of safety looks like. How do we get there?

How to Do It

How do we transform the dysfunctional cultures of health-care organizations into cultures of safety? How do we motivate CEOs to make safety a priority, take responsibility for making it happen, inspire others to join the cause, and create an environment of transparency, respect, and personal responsibility?

The leading thought leaders in patient safety have described visions of what a safe culture should be but often have been humble about providing advice on how to get there.

Reason speaks of "engineering" a safe culture in general, not specifically in health care. He describes the critical subcomponents: a reporting culture, a just culture, a flexible culture, and a learning culture. He notes that a safety culture is far more than the sum of its parts, that the rest is "up to the organizational chemistry" [8]. How to create that chemistry is left unanswered.

Likewise, Vincent describes the ingredients in a safety culture and notes that the evidence from studies such as those of Singer [19] shows that a better safety climate is associated with fewer adverse events. But he, too, shies away from prescribing how to achieve a safe culture [7].

However, in their perceptive and influential book, *Safer Healthcare: Strategies for the Real World*, Vincent and Amalberti provide a prescription for achieving safe care that would, in fact, require significant culture change [20]. They observe that the approach to improving patient safety has been too limited, focusing primarily on hospital care and too little on primary care and home care, and that the method used was the same in all settings: improvement of a core issue in a narrow time scale with a specific process change such as the surgical checklist or CLABSI protocol.

They call for a much broader approach using five safety strategies:

1. *Safety as Best Practice*: aspire to standards—reducing specific harms and improving clinical processes, such as the CLABSI protocol and the surgical checklist
2. *Improvement of Healthcare Processes and Systems*: intervening to support individuals and teams, improving working conditions and organizational practices, such as improved handovers, use of daily goals and huddles, and barcoding of medications
3. *Risk Control*: placing restrictions on performance, demand, or working conditions, such as regulations governing radiation therapy, closing unsafe facilities, and limiting individual licenses or privileges
4. *Improving Capacity for Monitoring, Adaptation, and Response*, such as briefings and debriefings, safe reporting, family engagement, and emergency planning
5. *Mitigation*: planning for potential harm and recovery, such as providing patient and peer support after harm

They then show how these five strategies can be used in three settings: hospital, home, and primary care. The specific issue of changing the culture to enable implementation of these strategies is not addressed, however.

Shanafelt et al. are more prescriptive [21]. They describe the steps that must be taken to change the culture of medicine: create psychological safety for people to learn new things, identify collaborative strategies for physicians and leaders to gain experience with new modes of working, and provide resources and formal training, advisors, and coaching. They emphasize that the leader must be convinced of the need to change and spearhead and support the initiatives. Individuals who are the targets of the change must be involved in the process [21].

IHI/Safe and Reliable Healthcare Framework   In 2017, the IHI and Safe and Reliable Healthcare jointly published *A Framework for Safe, Reliable, and Effective Care* [9]. The authors, Allan Frankel, cofounder of Safe and Reliable Healthcare, and Carol Haraden, Frank Federico, and Jennifer Lenoci-Edwards, of IHI, propose that achieving safe and reliable care requires attention to three domains: leadership, culture, and the learning system.

The paper provides direction to health-care organizations on the key strategic, clinical, operational, and cultural components involved with each and how they interact. It provides definitions and implementation strategies for nine foundational components: leadership, psychological safety, accountability, teamwork and communication, negotiation, transparency, reliability, improvement and measurement, and continuous learning.

Each of the nine components is described with specific major points, followed by a section, Moving from Concept to Reality, which describes the steps to implementing the ideas in daily practice. For example, the Framework uses Edmondson's definition of psychological safety [22]:

- Anyone can ask questions without looking stupid.
- Anyone can ask for feedback without looking incompetent.
- Anyone can be respectfully critical without appearing negative.
- Anyone can suggest innovative ideas without being perceived as disruptive.

It then gives advice on how to achieve psychological safety, such as coaching, huddles, solicitation of ideas, and providing feedback to suggestions. As the authors suggest, the report provides a framework for thinking about patient safety; training, guidance, and support are also needed. It is not a blueprint or detailed plan.

ACHE/LLI Leading a Culture of Safety   That blueprint is provided for the key element for culture change, leadership, by another publication in 2017, *Leading a Culture of Safety: A Blueprint for Success*, jointly published by the American College of Healthcare Executives and the Lucian Leape Institute [23]. The most detailed and prescriptive advice published so far, its central theme is that leaders create safety. The product of two roundtables of those who have led and those who have studied successful transformations, the document is "an evidence-based, practical resource with tools and proven strategies to assist (leaders) in creating a culture of safety" [23].

The mission is clearly stated up front: "It is both the obligation and the privilege of every healthcare CEO to create and represent a compelling vision for a culture of safety: a culture in which mistakes are acknowledged and lead to sustainable, positive change; respectful and inclusive behaviors are instinctive and serve as the behavioral norms for the organization; and the physical and psychological safety of patients and the workforce is both highly valued and ardently protected…. The elimination of harm to our patients and workforce is our foremost moral and ethical obligation" [23].

The document addresses both "foundational" elements—what is needed to establish a culture of safety—and "sustaining" elements, what is needed to make it permanent. It describes in detail the many elements of both strategy and tactics that are needed to accomplish the objectives. These are organized into six leadership domains that require CEO focus and dedication:

1. *Establish a compelling vision for safety*. An organization's vision reflects priorities that, when aligned with its mission, establish a strong foundation for the work of the organization.
2. *Build trust, respect, and inclusion*. Establishing trust, showing respect, and promoting inclusion—and demonstrating these principles throughout the organization and with patients and families—are essential to a leader's ability to create and sustain a culture of safety.
3. *Select, develop, and engage your Board*. CEOs are responsible for ensuring the education of their Board members on foundational safety science.

4. *Prioritize safety in the selection and development of leaders.* Include accountability for safety as part of the leadership development strategy for the organization. In addition, identify physicians, nurses, and other clinical leaders as safety champions.
5. *Lead and reward a just culture.* Workers must be empowered and unafraid to voice concerns about threats to patient and workforce safety.
6. *Establish organizational behavior expectations.* These include transparency, effective teamwork, active communication, civility, and direct and timely feedback.

Leading a Culture of Safety is a landmark publication. It is by far the most comprehensive exposition of what is needed to achieve a safe culture in health care. It is a blueprint constructed by the most respected leaders in the field that makes a clear and powerful statement that the trust and openness needed to achieve a safe culture start at the top.

Examples of Success

A handful of health-care organizations have succeeded in changing their cultures. Several are worth examining for lessons learned.

Virginia Mason Medical Center

In 2000, Virginia Mason Medical Center (VMMC) in Seattle was in trouble. It was losing money, and it became apparent that the old model based on professional excellence was insufficient. The Board and top management had all read the IOM reports and realized that they too had quality and safety problems and inefficiencies. The Board asked, "if we are so focused on patients, why are all the systems built around the doctors?" Agreeing, Gary Kaplan, the new CEO, proposed to change from a physician-driven organization focused on volume to a patient-oriented organization based on quality of care. The Board gave him full support.

Kaplan and his senior management team spent the next year looking unsuccessfully for a health-care management system to achieve this goal. They then accidentally met John Black, a former Boeing executive, who told them of the impact of implementing the management system Lean. They visited businesses in the USA that used Lean and decided it was what they needed.

Lean is derived from the Toyota Production System that was developed in the 1930s when Toyota began producing automobiles [24]. It is founded on the concept of continuous and incremental improvements of product and process and eliminating waste. It is "a way to do more and more with less and less - less human effort, less equipment, less time, and less space - while coming closer and closer to providing customers exactly what they want" [25].

Lean is based on five key principles:

1. *Value*: Specify the value desired by the customer.
2. *Value Stream*: Identify the *value stream* (*the steps in a process*) that provides value for each product, and challenge all of the wasted steps.
3. *Flow*: Make the product flow continuously through the remaining value-added steps.
4. *Pull*: Introduce pull between all steps where continuous flow is possible.
5. *Perfection*: Manage toward perfection so that the number of steps and the amount of time and information needed to serve the customer continually fall [26].

Persuaded by Black and Carolyn Corvi, who had led dramatic improvements in the production of the 737 aircraft, Kaplan took his senior executive team to Japan to study the Toyota Production System. They were profoundly moved. Workers and managers worked in harmony to produce a flawless product, an automobile. Kaplan's team could see that these methods could be adapted to health care. They came home determined to develop a Virginia Mason Production System (VMPS).

Aren't You Ashamed? One experience at Toyota struck home with particular force. A *sensei* (teacher) reviewing a VMMC floor plan with the team asked what a certain area was. A waiting room, they said. "Who waits there?" Patients. "For whom?" The doctor. The sensei then found that there were 100 waiting rooms at VMMC and that patients waited on average 45 minutes for a doctor. "Aren't you ashamed?" he said [27]. Suddenly the team understood what "patient first" meant.

Back home, selling VMPS to the staff was another matter. While many—particularly the younger ones who had embraced quality improvement—were supportive, some of the senior staff, including some department chairmen, were not. They rebelled, objected, and in some cases resigned. Education about the new system and training leaders took a year or more, but it was imperative, and the investment of time proved worthwhile.

The changes proposed were indeed monumental. It took several years to implement them, and the work is never done. Four features drove the transformation:

1. A *shared vision* outlined within a strategic plan that places the *Patient First* in everything, always. The strategic plan evolved into a "pyramid" figure with the patient at the top; under that, the vision and the mission; and then the values teamwork, integrity, excellence, and service.
2. *Alignment* of mission and values from the board down. Alignment means all parties share common focus, common goal, common language, and common culture. The "pyramid" facilitates alignment—there is no ambiguity that the patient's interest is always first.

   A key instrument for achieving alignment is the *compact*, an agreement between the organization and physicians that made explicit the reciprocal obligations of both. It took a year to develop. Additional compacts were developed for leaders and for board members.
3. A single improvement *method*—VMPS—that enables continuing improvements in quality, safety, access, efficiency, and affordability, every day at every level of the organization.
4. A culture predicated on deep respect for people and continuous improvement. Two aspects are fundamental: *respect*, meaning every voice is not only heard, but listened to, and *teamwork* that stimulates personal and professional growth and performance.

The transformations of the VMPS were many and profound. They have been extensively documented and explained in several books that are well worth reading [27–29].

Here are a few examples:

Standard Work   A challenge for physicians was the concept of standard work, a cornerstone of innovation in Lean. Reducing variability ensures quality while making it easier to identify and deal with necessary exceptions. Standard work means that all have the obligation to follow a process that is defined by consensus among stakeholders as the most effective and safest. Embracing this concept was an essential first step in establishing the new culture. Over the years, VMMC developed over 70 "must do" processes.

Kaizen Promotion Office (KPO)   "Kaizen" is Japanese for continuous incremental improvement. It assumes that frontline workers are the source of ideas of how to remove waste and improve processes but lack the expertise to develop the new processes. Expert help is needed. At VMMC, the KPO provides that help. The KPO was a clear signal that VMMC was serious about VMPS.

Rapid Process Improvement Workshops (RPIW)   One of the earliest innovations introduced was the Rapid Process Improvement Workshop. This is an intensely serious effort to address a defined quality or flow problem. Trained and certified Workshop leaders convene a team of stakeholders and KPO experts to work full time for 5 days to analyze a problem, identify waste, define the value stream, and reengineer the process. Stretch goals are set—typically 50% for operational issues, 100% for safety.

Examples of innovation from RPIWs include eliminating the waiting rooms in outpatient clinics, cutting triage time in the ER in half, and the institution of Saturday hours. A powerful example was redesigning the cancer center, which took multiple RPIWs.

When VMMC decided to move the cancer center to a large floor with windows all around the periphery, the doctors assumed that is where their offices would be. Not so. If VMMC was serious about putting the patient's interest first, they would go to the patients. And so it was, with the doctors and nurses having their offices and common areas internally.

Not only did the patients get the nice rooms, they could stay there. Analysis of the "value stream" showed that cancer patients typically spent hours walking all over the hospital to see multiple specialists;

get X-rays, lab tests; etc., in addition to lying in bed for hours for intravenous infusion. The fix? A truly radical idea: let them stay in the room and have everyone come to them. Result: the duration of patient visits fell by 50%, patient satisfaction rose to 95%, and VMMC took care of 1100 more patients a year with no increase in staff [27].

Patient Safety Alerts (PSA) Safe and frequent reporting of errors, adverse events, near misses, and hazards is essential to improvement. You can't fix something you don't know about. VMMC labelled them Patient Safety Alerts (PSA) and patterned the response after Toyota's "Stop the Line." Mishaps were no longer "events" to be reported and perhaps evaluated, they were real-time indicators of failure and harm and got immediate attention.

Two features distinguish the PSA system from the usual reporting system: everyone is empowered and obligated to report them in real time, and every report leads to a response. The response may be immediate, stopping a treatment to correct or understand an error or near miss, or urgent root cause analysis, or as an agenda item for improvement. The PSA system enables the frontline worker to directly engage leadership in a collaborative relationship. It is also tangible evidence of the institution's commitment to the target of perfection.

Since its inception in 2002, the PSA system has resulted in 100,000 reports that led to responses and changes that over time dramatically reduced the rate of adverse events and "near misses." Risk-adjusted mortality declined, as did liability costs.

Patient Safety as a Primary Goal In 2004, Mary McClinton died at VMMC during a radiological procedure as a result of accidental intravenous injection of an antiseptic, chlorhexidine, instead of contrast material. The hospital was devastated. Unequivocally committed to transparency, Kaplan went public, explained what happened, and apologized. The newspapers remarked on how unusual his transparency was (and, sadly, still is).

Mary McClinton's death had a profound impact on the hospital staff. In the previous two years, they had made great strides in improving processes and reducing errors. How could this happen? Clearly, they still had a long way to go to achieve harm-free care. But the experience with improving quality and the development of a culture of openness and trust gave them confidence to proceed. The response was quick and decisive: patient safety would not just be part of the transformation, it would become its overarching goal. Prevention of harm would be the core focus for the next several years.

Respect for People In 2011, after a decade of incredibly successful cultural transformation, a routine survey showed that, like other health-care organizations, nearly half of employees still did not feel safe in speaking up about a personal mistake. Lynne Chafez, General Counsel and leader of the changes at VMMC, asked me to come out and consult with them.

We had just written our papers on respect (Chap. 21), so I shared our discovery of the unrecognized subtle forms of disrespect that are pervasive in health care. It fell on fertile ground. They listened, and they responded by developing the Respect for People program as a major safety goal. VMMC developed an educational course on respect that was required for all 5000 of their staff. The approach has subsequently been adopted by hundreds of other hospitals worldwide. It identified ten foundational behaviors expected of everyone working at VMMC. They speak volumes about the kind of culture it strives to be (Box 23.1).

Box 23.1 Respect for People
Foundational behaviors

1. Listen to understand
2. Keep your promises
3. Be encouraging
4. Connect with others
5. Express gratitude
6. Share information
7. Speak up
8. Walk in their shoes
9. Grow and develop
10. Be a team player

Adapted from Ref. [28].

Secrets of Success

The transformation of VMMC was a profound and dramatic culture change. It was challenging, it was threatening, and it never stops. Reflecting on 18 years of progress, Gary Kaplan identified four key transformations that led to successful culture change:

First, *Board and governance engagement*. Members of the board are responsible for governance, not just to attend meetings and leave quality to the doctors, but as partners to achieve it. Board members are trained in VMPS, and, like all senior leaders, every member of the Board is required to go to Japan at least once in their first term. They undergo regular self-evaluation as a board and as individuals.

The Board is seriously involved in ensuring patient respect and care. Patient care failures and successes are presented at every meeting, sometimes by the patient in person. The Board reviews every red PSA (an event that has harmed a patient or has the potential to) and must sign off on the prevention plan before it is implemented.

Clearly, it is a very different kind of board from those of most health-care organizations. Members are neither appointed by CEO nor beholden to him. They are chosen for their expertise, literacy and commitment, not their status in the community or largess. They bring curiosity, active engagement and dissent in open meetings, and, as defined in their compact, relentless commitment to the strategic plan. Outside experts such as Julie Morath and Gregg Meyer are included on the oversight committee.

Second, Kaplan believes *changing minds of leadership* is crucial. All members of the "C-suite"—including legal counsel and the CFO—have to become champions to support middle management. Trust, alignment, and workers' sense of value depend on leadership. Trust comes from leaders being vulnerable in the sense of being willing to admit mistakes and take advice from others. Alignment depends on leaders who are value-driven, embrace the mission and the strategic plan, and have clarity about purpose. Alignment to purpose and respect for people gives workers passion about their work and meaning to their lives.

Continuing development of new leaders is the key to sustainability. VMMC has an active program to continually identify, develop, and formally train leaders at all levels. One or two people are always prepared to step up when someone leaves.

The third critical transformation is *transparency*—truth telling—shining a light on mistakes. Transparency creates the culture that makes reporting work; it reveals behaviors that are not consistent with *patient first*. It ensures open and honest communication with patients when things go wrong. A culture of transparency revealed the problem of disrespect. External transparency, as in the McClinton's, builds trust with the public.

Finally, the fourth transformation is the centerpiece *respect for people*, listening and responding to staff concerns and holding all accountable for respectful conduct with one another and with patients.

VMMC is a model of the transformation needed for a health-care organization to develop a culture of safety. Safety is an organizing principle of its daily work, a pillar supporting its mission to provide high-quality effective care. Zero harm is the goal, safety is everyone's responsibility, and innovation and improvement are part of everyday work. Not surprisingly, year after year, VMMC has been named as one of the top hospitals in the nation by Leapfrog. Hundreds of health-care organizations have come to VMMC to learn how to transform. May they all succeed.

Cincinnati Children's Hospital

When Jim Anderson took over as CEO at Cincinnati Children's Hospital (CCH) in 1997, he found a hospital that, like most academic institutions of the time, prided itself on its research excellence and assumed that its patient care was excellent as well. Anderson was not so sure. Having been CEO of a manufacturing firm, he knew something about quality improvement, and he knew CCH could do better. Lee Carter, the new board chair agreed. He was especially interested in increasing the focus on patients and families.

In 1999, they initiated a strategic planning process that asked their various communities about challenges over the next 3–5 years. One of the groups said that despite having great physicians and nurses, the institution did not provide an environment for the best delivery of that care.

There was more disturbing news. CCH had just joined the Cystic Fibrosis Foundation (CFF) National Quality Initiative, a collaborative with other hospitals to improve the care of cystic fibrosis patients. When they received comparative feedback of baseline data of measures of nutrition and pulmonary function, they were shocked to find that CCH was not only not in the top 10 as they expected, but its results were below the national average.

From his business experience, Anderson knew that fixing quality problems was not only the right thing to do, but that the savings more than offset the costs, making also a compelling business case. Poor quality came from inept management. Carter agreed. They could do better.

The release of the IOM report, *To Err is Human*, provided additional impetus. Quality and safety were compelling issues they needed to address. CCH's new 5-year strategic plan made a commitment to dramatically transform the way they delivered health care. Uma Kotagal, who had led earlier performance efforts, was put in charge.

Lee Carter's comment was memorable: "Well, if we are not the best, we can certainly be the best at getting better, and then we *will* be the best." He established and chaired the Board Patient Care Committee, composed of doctors, nurses, business people, board members, and members of the community.

In the middle of the strategic planning process came the opportunity to apply for a Pursuing Perfection grant from the Robert Wood Johnson Foundation (RWJF) (see Chap. 6 for program details). CCH competed against over 200 hospitals and was one of only four chosen. They would focus on one evidence-based practice, bronchiolitis, and one chronic condition, cystic fibrosis, which they knew from the national quality initiative they needed to work on. After a struggle with CFF, they obtained the name of the hospital that was the national leader in cystic fibrosis care and sent a team to learn from them how to improve their care of these patients.

A core requirement of the RWJF grant was transparency and patient engagement. The Foundation funded and helped produce a video of CCH parents of patients with cystic fibrosis who volunteered to describe their experiences. The film was devastating. It depicted multiple errors in the care they were receiving. Anderson showed it to the Board Patient Care Committee. They were speechless, except for the doctors or nurses who said, "Of course, that's how the system works." Anderson and Kotagal had their work cut out for them.

Participating in Pursuing Perfection had a powerful impact on CCH. While it yielded impressive successes, it also revealed how far they had to go to build capacity to make widespread change. Kotagal realized that people didn't know how to make change. They needed to be trained. She sent key staff to take Brent James' QI course in Salt Lake City.

A central feature of the reorganization was the establishment of clinical systems improvement (CSI) teams consisting of a physician leader, a nurse leader, and executive for each of five domains: inpatient, outpatient, perioperative, home health, and emergency. These CSI teams were responsible for major issues such as flow, safety, and patient experience. They worked with and sponsored unit teams headed by a physician leader and the nurse manager to test patient safety initiatives. All were required to take the course on leadership and capability development.

A robust measurement system was developed to document outcomes, and within each domain influential physicians and nurses formed improvement teams for key negative outcomes such as ventilator-associated pneumonia, catheter-associated bloodstream infections, surgical site infections, and adverse drug events. A senior leader was assigned as champion for each team. Families were involved as members of the teams. Stretch goals were set and met.

Significant improvements occurred and were sustained. As they increased QI capability and developed knowledge of reliability design, they were able to further improve and simultaneously carry out dozens of improvements and build systems capable of 95–99% reliability.

Nonetheless, in 2005 the organization realized its rate of sentinel or serious safety events (SSE) was still high. With the help of consultants, it decided to change the safety management system to apply HRO concepts. They developed five key drivers to achieve a goal of reducing the SSE rate by 80% over 3 years:

1. Restructured governance for patient safety
2. Developing a highly reliable error prevention system
3. A transparent culture of continuous learning

4. State-of-the-art detection and cause analysis system
5. Focused intervention on perioperative processes and culture

Senior leaders adopted Patient Safety as the core value of the organization, and a commitment was made to change the culture by changing behavior. All frontline staff were trained on key safety behaviors, reinforced daily via safety coaches. An organization-wide focus on "Days since the last SSE" continuously gave a sense of wariness and unease. SSE were reduced by 65% in 3 years.

A rigorous root cause analysis process was implemented, overseen by the legal department to ensure that it was a trusted process that everyone could believe in. Senior executives were accountable to make sure it happened in timely way. They took ownership of the problem. This led the staff to have confidence in the process and accept transparency.

In 2005, Cincinnati Children's Hospital, now called Cincinnati Children's Hospital Medical Center (CCHMC), partnered with the other children's hospitals in Ohio and the Ohio Children's Hospital Association to improve safety. The first effort was implementation of medical response teams in all of the hospitals. Cardiopulmonary arrests outside of intensive care units were reduced by 46%. As Kotagal's successor, Steve Muething, recalled, this was a "game changer" for CCHMC: they realized that they could improve better and have more influence by working with others.

Under the leadership of Muething and the new CEO, Michael Fisher, and with funding from CMS and private industry, CCHMC joined the other Ohio children's hospitals in 2009 to formalize this collaboration for safety as the Ohio Children's Hospitals' Solutions for Patient Safety network. Hospital personnel were trained in the Model for Improvement and shared lessons learned with one another. ADEs were subsequently reduced by 50% and SSIs in high-risk children by 60% in all eight hospitals.

In 2012, 25 hospitals across the nation joined the initial 8 Ohio hospitals to form Solutions for Patient Safety (SPS), a network that eventually grew to 142 children's hospitals collaborating to reduce serious patient harm. From 2011 to 2018, hospitals in the SPS reduced their adverse drug events by 74%, catheter-associated urinary infections by 50%, falls by 75%, and pressure ulcers by 27%.

Kotagal and Muething attribute CCHMC's success to six factors:

1. *Alignment and commitment.* From the beginning, Anderson, Carter, and Kotagal were clear and unambiguous about the focus and led the board, senior leaders, and CSI chairs to share a deep commitment to zero serious harm, leadership improvement, and partnerships between physicians and nurses and between leaders and researchers.
2. *Structure for change and integration.* The creation of Clinical System Improvement teams of top leaders for each of the major delivery systems gave coherence and clear responsibility for major changes to improve flow, processes, and patient experience. They worked with unit teams led by trained physician and nurse leaders who carried out specific projects, aligning macro-, meso-, and microsystem structure across the entire system. Patient safety and staff safety were integrated.
3. *Capability and capacity for change.* From the beginning, the organization invested deeply in training in the science of improvement and in the infrastructure support, analytics, and operational research needed to create good visibility of data, response, and action.
4. *Creation of a culture of continuous learning.* Creation of psychological safety, the opportunities for constant improvement, and training in leadership and quality improvement created an environment where learning is part of everyday life.
5. *Respect for the Science.* The belief in the scientific approach enabled the organization to be rational and logical and attract very bright people with a passion to do well by children.
6. *Transparency.* A culture where it is normal and expected that people will surface, address, and ultimately solve issues/problems every day at all levels, especially when things go wrong, is the foundation of trust. Adverse events were promptly acknowledged to the staff, patients, and the public, thoroughly investigated, and the results fed back to the family and to the clinical staff for improvement.

Cincinnati Children's Hospital Medical Center has truly created a culture of safety. It has developed, and continues to refine, a sustainable model of collaborative patient and staff engagement in continuing improvement that has dramatically reduced harm for its patients. It has stimulated other children's hospitals to change their cultures and collaborated with them to do so. They are an impressive model.

Denver Health

Denver Health (DH) is an example of an apparently impressive culture change that turned out to be illusory. Denver Health is the principal safety-net provider in Colorado, providing health care for nearly a third of Denver's population, 46% of whom are uninsured. In 2004, under the leadership of its CEO, Patricia Gabow, MD, and with a grant from AHRQ, DH began a major initiative to transform the way it delivered care, centered on five "Rights":

- Right People: a workforce committed to customer service and quality
- Right Environment: appropriate patient and work spaces
- Right Reward for employees who demonstrate customer-oriented behaviors
- Right Communication and Culture
- Right Process: application of Lean to eliminate waste

Gabow created a new department to take responsibility for patient safety and quality and focus on processes to improve care. Programs were created to manage high-risk and high-opportunity clinical situations, such as failure to rescue, use of antibiotics, CLABSI, etc. Systems were implemented to reduce variability in patient care processes and outcomes. The initiative was supported by a sophisticated electronic health record that provided order entry and decision support in addition to data for research and quality improvement [30].

Like VMMC, Denver Health developed an intensive approach to process change, the Rapid Improvement Event (RIE), a four-day group session focused on an identified problem to develop a method to remove it. Rapid improvement events resulted in marked advances in diabetes care, anticoagulation management, venous thromboembolism prophylaxis, and cancer screening rates.

In its first 4 years, DH estimated that it also gained $42 million in financial benefit due to reduced waste. In 2009, it had the lowest observed/expected aggregate mortality ratio among 106 academic health centers in the University HealthSystem Consortium. Denver Health was hailed as an impressive example of rapid and effective culture change.

Gabow retired in 2012, having received numerous awards and honors for her impressive work at transforming a health-care organization. In 2014, she told her story in *The Lean Prescription: Powerful Medicine for Our Ailing Healthcare System*, which she wrote with Philip Goodman [31].

Then it came undone. Gabow was succeeded by Arthur Gonzales, who quickly undid many of Gabow's changes in response to financial pressures associated with the Affordable Care Act. His leadership style alienated physicians and led to resignations of a number of physicians, including all of the chairs of the major departments. Gonzales was later replaced by Robin Wittenstein.

The rapid reversal of the culture at Denver Health illustrates the difficulty of making real culture change that is sustainable. The impressive transformations implemented by Gabow were evidently not institutionalized well enough among the executive leaders, employees, and middle managers to withstand a change of top leadership. The culture really didn't change. And one can infer that the board was not totally engaged in the transformation and lacked continuity of purpose, or it would not have hired a CEO who put financial goals over safety.

Safe and Reliable Health Care

On a national scale, the most comprehensive effort to date to change culture by developing organizational capacity and capability is a proprietary effort developed by Safe and Reliable Healthcare (S&R), the consulting firm established by Allan Frankel and Michael Leonard, two highly respected physicians who have devoted their professional careers to improving patient safety. Frankel was for years the chief patient safety officer for Partners Healthcare in Boston and on the faculty at IHI. Leonard was for many years the chief safety officer at Kaiser-Permanente.

S&R trains a health-care organization's leadership and its personnel to create and sustain the environment for safe care. The focus of the S&R method is to give frontline personnel *voice* and a *sense of community*. Voice, or agency, means that everyone feels safe to speak up and that their voice is heard and respected and influences what takes place. Community means that everyone feels that their co-workers care about them. The S&R approach changes the structure of the management of the delivery of care and improvement so that voice and community are intrinsic to everyday work.

The following description is adapted from the S&R website [32]:

The core of the S&R approach is a digital platform called LENS™ (*Learning and ENgagement System*), an interactive electronic replacement of the white board where staff gather daily to define issues, develop plans, receive updates, celebrate achievements, and recognize contributions. It enables physical and virtual rounds, huddles, and improvement work so that leaders and managers can effectively communicate and visibly "close the loop" on ideas and concerns shared by frontline teams. This enables real-time coordination and improvement as well as alignment and coordination within a unit and collaboration across multiple teams. Frontline teams have "voice, visibility, and ownership" in shaping their unit's culture and performance.

A key element is SCORE, a system that obtains survey data and provides analysis to support LENS. It builds on and expands the earlier surveys of patients and providers developed by Sexton, AHRQ, and others but differs by being correlated with outcomes based on data from over 700 organizations. SCORE includes questions on culture, engagement, burnout, resilience, patient experience, physician satisfaction, and Magnet. It maps to AHRQ/SOPS, SAQ, and other surveys, thus enabling use of previous data to benchmark and show

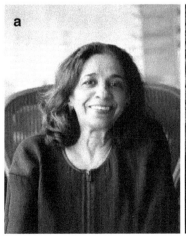
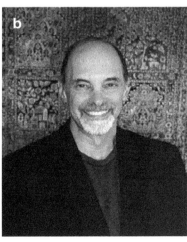
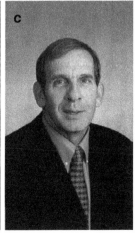

(**a**) Uma Kotagal, (**b**) Allan Frankel, and (**c**) Mike Leonard. (All rights reserved)

improvement. Data are presented graphically and automated to show unit results and trends across the organization.

S&R team of experts provides guidance for becoming a high-reliability organization. The goal is to generate organizational capacity and a sustainable architecture for excellence by empowering leaders, managers, and teams to clearly understand what they must measure and improve across their transformation journey. The S&R approach holds great promise. It seeks to change the culture by changing behavior at all levels. To the extent that includes engaging top management and the boards in the transformation, the changes should be sustained.

As of this writing, 12 systems of care, representing dozens of hospitals and hundreds of care units, are working with S&R to create safe and cost-effective health care. Time will tell if they succeed.

Making It Happen

What will it take to get hospitals and health-care systems nationwide to implement the VMMC, CCHMC, or S&R models to make the transformations needed to change their cultures? As the experiences of VMMC and CCHMC show, the CEO must have the vision and skills to make it happen and the passion and commitment to carry through. The Board must share that commitment and provide the resources and the backup when the going gets tough.

Perhaps exposure to advanced thinking about leadership, quality, and patient safety, such as by the initiative of the ACHE, combined with increasing evidence of success by peer health-care organizations, will motivate more leaders of organizations to "do the right thing."

But the motives of others engaged in reform may be less high-minded. For a decade or so, CEOs have been bombarded by a stream of articles in the Harvard Business Review and elsewhere about the power of Reliability Science to improve efficiency, including occasional examples in health care. They are beginning to realize that managing the complexity of care demands standardization and simplification of services and that these changes require employee engagement.

So, to be financially sound and deliver safe care, they have joined the trend to embrace reliability science and Lean. The "in" thing is to become an HRO. Many major health-care organizations now have a process engineering office and black belt leaders. The employee focus has advanced from satisfaction to engagement, resilience, and wellness. Resistance to change has lessened as the fraction of younger physicians has increased and the values of autonomy and hierarchy are being replaced by cooperation, teamwork, and respect.

This is an encouraging trend, but there is a dark side. The major trend is directed at the bottom line: consolidation. In our profit-oriented fee-for-service health-care system, market share is everything. Across the country, the big guys are swallowing up the little guys. Some are long-standing, national in scope, and huge, such as HCA (186 hospitals), Ascension Health (151), and Trinity Health (104), and span large geographic areas. Others, such as MGH Brigham (14) in Boston and Northwell (23) in Long Island, are expanding regional monopolies. Others are doing the same thing.

The primary objective of consolidation is financial success. National systems implement standardized practices to increase profits by improving efficiency and reducing costs. Regional monopolies also seek to eliminate competition in order to guarantee market share and raise prices.

In fairness, it is important to note that some large consolidated systems have been leaders in quality improvement and safety. In the current milieu, they can be an effective way to spread systems changes such as Lean and worker engagement. We have the "Ascension Way," the "Trinity Way," etc. that, when well directed, can result in significant changes.

Nonetheless, in most systems, the CFO keeps management focused on the bottom line. The demand for productivity and profits competes with quality and safety, and usually wins, as evidenced by the high burnout rates among physicians and nurses in many of these hospitals. Safety is not the primary goal.

A Role for Government?

So the big question is what will it take to get all hospital CEOs and Boards motivated to make the culture change we need to make care safe and efficient? To make patient safety "job one"? There is no clear answer, but several possibilities come to mind.

One would be federal oversight. Congress could create an FAA equivalent for health care, a Federal Patient Safety Agency, FPSA, to set standards and monitor and enforce compliance. In addition to setting standards for physician competence as described in Chap. 20, the Agency would develop standards for all aspects of health-care delivery in collaboration with representatives from hospitals and health-care systems, the Joint Commission, professional societies, and experts in quality and safety. As noted earlier, participation by stakeholders in developing standards ensures relevance and buy-in with a higher likelihood of compliance.

Specifically for safety, the Agency would set standards for practice, including training in quality and safety, data collection, working conditions, coordination of care, transparency, and reporting. It would require reporting of all serious reportable events. Failure to report would have consequences, such as prohibiting reimbursement of a hospital for any charges for an admission with a SRE. Repeat offenders could be fined and face loss of accreditation.

Given the current political climate, indeed, the climate of the past several decades, it seems highly unlikely there would be Congressional support for significantly increased regulation. A lesser measure, such as requiring *enterprise liability* in which the health-care organization is held accountable for a patient injury rather than the physician, might be possible and would be useful, but also seems unlikely.

Can nongovernmental oversight, such as by the Joint Commission, provide sufficient pressure to motivate health-care organizations to change their cultures? Perhaps. Over the past few years, the Joint Commission has steadily increased requirements for accreditation to promote quality and safety, including implementation of safe practices, reporting of SRE, adherence to core measures of quality, ensuring physician competence, patient engagement, and assessment of patient experience. (See Chap. 12.) Joint Commission Patient Safety Goals have been internalized by many hospitals. These measures have had an impact on the cultures.

However, the ability of the Joint Commission to expand its requirements is limited by its vulnerability to competition. CMS also accepts accreditation of hospitals by other organizations to receive the essential "deemed status" that enables them to receive payments from Medicare and Medicaid. Because these alternative programs are less demanding, they are an attractive "way out" if TJC gets too tough. This could, of course, be turned around if CMS gave the Commission sole accrediting authority, subject to CMS oversight.

A "Burning Platform"?

Some believe that health-care organizations will not change in the absence of an existential threat, a "burning platform." That our dysfunctional system has to get worse before it can get better. To really be threatening, that threat has to be financial.

Many, your author included, believe that the fundamental cause of the dysfunction of the American health-care system is the way hospitals and doctors are paid. The USA is the only advanced economy that runs health care as a business. That business is based on the fee-for-service (FFS) system for paying for health care. The primary goal of any business is to make a profit. In a fee-for-service system, the more services hospitals or doctors provide, the better they do.

The ramifications and nuances of this system are far too complex to be dealt with here, but the implications are clear: in a FFS payment system, the need to focus on productivity and profit is a major deterrent to hospitals making quality of care and patient safety their core mission. Changing to a risk-adjusted capitated system, such as an accountable care organization, with oversight to ensure that standards of appropriateness, quality, and safety are met, would give new meaning to the "bottom line." By itself, changing the payment system would not change the culture, but it would remove the major barrier and provide the right incentives.

Will the COVID-19 pandemic be the "burning platform" that forces change? Under its stress, our health-care system collapsed. Increasing demand for highly expensive COVID care, coupled with a decline in demand for routine services, led to crippling financial losses that have driven substantial numbers of hospitals and office practices into bankruptcy, especially rural and safety net hospitals. In our FFS business model, when markets collapse, so do providers [33].

The pandemic also significantly undermined the system of funding of health care for patients. Millions lost their employment-based health insurance when they lost their jobs [33]. Government subsidies were insufficient to make up for these losses.

As of this writing, it is impossible to know how things will turn out. However, the crisis has increased the national will for universal coverage and for insurance that is not work-related. A substantial majority of Americans now embrace the concept that health care should be a right. All of the approaches to achieve that goal require significant long-term federal outlays, as well as a huge infusion of funds short-term to prevent further collapse of the system.

Will this unprecedented requirement to fund coverage also lead to the recognition of the need to redesign the health-care system to eliminate unnecessary, harmful, and wasteful care? To design a system to meet patient needs, not to make money? Will it be what it takes to move Congress to change the financing of health care from fee-for-service to capitation, from for-profit care to patient-centered accountable care? Will this be what it takes to make patient safety a reality? If so, our suffering will not have been in vain.

References

1. Dixon-Woods M, Bosk CL, Aveling EL, et al. Explaining Michigan: developing an ex post theory of a quality improvement program. Milbank Q. 2011;89:167–205.
2. Leape LL. Error in medicine. JAMA. 1994;272:1851–7.
3. Kohn KT, Corrigan JM, Donaldson MS, editors. To err is human: building a safer health system. Washington: National Academy Press; 1999.
4. Schein EH. Organizational culture and leadership. 4th ed. San Francisco: Jossey-Bass; 2010.
5. Edwards JRD, Davey J, Armstrong K. Returning to the roots of culture: a review and re-conceptualisation of safety culture. Saf Sci. 2013;55:70–80.
6. Glendon AI, Stanton NA. Perspectives on safety culture. Saf Sci. 2000;34:193–214.
7. Vincent C. Patient safety. 2nd ed. Chichester: BMJ Books; 2010.
8. Reason JT. Managing the risks of organizational accidents. Aldershot, Hants; Brookfield: Ashgate; 1997.
9. Frankel A, Haraden C, Federico F, Lenoci-Edwards J. A framework for safe, reliable and effective care. White Paper: Institute for Healthcare Improvement; 2017.
10. Marx D. Patient safety and the "just culture": a primer for health care executives. New York. 17 Apr 2001.

11. Singer S, Lin S, Falwell A, Gaba D, Baker L. Relationship of safety climate and safety performance in hospitals. Health Serv Res. 2009;44:399–421.
12. Roberts KH. New challenges to organizational research: high reliability organizations. Ind Crisis Q. 1989;3:111–25.
13. Weick KE, Sutcliffe KM, Obstfeld D. Organizing for high reliability. Res Organ Behav. 1999;21:81–123.
14. Chassin MR, Loeb JM. The ongoing quality improvement journey: next stop, high reliability. Health Aff. 2011;30:559–68.
15. Roberts K, Stout S, Halpern J. Decision dynamics in two high reliability military organizations. Man Sci. 1994;40:614–24.
16. Institute of Medicine (US) Committee on Quality of Health Care in America. Crossing the quality chasm: a new health system for the 21st century. Washington: National Academies Press; 2001.
17. Top U.S. "Non-profit" hospitals & CEOs are racking up huge profits. 26 June 2019. Accessed October 3, 2020, at https://www.forbes.com/sites/ada-mandrzejewski/2019/06/26/top-u-s-non-profit-hospitals-ceos-are-racking-up-huge-profits/#33444d019dfb.
18. Leape LL, Berwick DM. Five years after "to err is human", what have we learned? JAMA. 2005;293:2384–90.
19. Singer SJ, Falwell A, Gaba DM, et al. Identifying organizational cultures that promote patient safety. Health Care Manag Rev. 2009;34:300–11.
20. Vincent C, Amalberti R. Safer healthcare: strategies for the real world. Cham: Springer; 2016.
21. Shanafelt TD, Schein E, Minor LB, Trockel M, Schein P, Kirch D. Healing the professional culture of medicine. Mayo Clin Proc. 2019;94:1556–66.
22. Edmondson AC. Psychological safety, trust, and learning in organizations: a group-level Lens. In: Kramer R, Cook K, editors. Trust and distrust in organizations: dilemmas and approaches. New York: Russell Sage Foundation; 2004. p. 239–72.
23. American College of Healthcare Executives and IHI/NPSF Lucian Leape Institute. Leading a culture of safety: a blueprint for success. Boston: American College of Healthcare Executives and Institute for Healthcare Improvement; 2017.
24. Ohno T, Bodek N. Toyota production system: beyond large-scale production. 1st ed. Portland: CRC Press; 1988.
25. Rizzardo D, Brooks R. Understanding Lean Manufacturing: Maryland Technology Enterprise Institute; 2003.
26. Womack JP, Jones DT. Lean thinking. 2nd ed. New York: Simon & Schuster, Inc.; 2003.
27. Kenney C. Transforming health care: Virginia Mason Medical Center's pursuit of the perfect patient experience. Boca Raton: CRC Press; 2011.
28. Kenney C. A leadership journey in health care: Virginia Mason's story. London: CRC Press; 2015.

29. Plsek PE. Accelerating health care transformation with lean and innovation: the Virginia Mason experience. Boca Raton: CRC Press; 2014.
30. Gabow PA, Mehler PS. A broad and structured approach to improving patient safety and quality: lessons from Denver Health. Health Aff. 2011;30:612–8.
31. Gabow PA, Goodman PL. The lean prescription: powerful medicine for our ailing healthcare system. Boca Raton: Productivity Press; 2015.
32. Safe & Reliable Healthcare. Accessed 3 Oct 2020, at https://safeandreliablecare.com/.
33. Blumenthal D, Fowler EJ, Abrams M, Collins SR. Covid-19 — implications for the health care system. N Engl J Med. 2020;383:1483–8.

Permissions

We would like to thank the editorial team for lending their expertise to make the book truly unique. They have played a crucial role in the development of this book. Without their invaluable contributions this book wouldn't have been possible. They have made vital efforts to compile up to date information on the varied aspects of this subject to make this book a valuable addition to the collection of many professionals and students.

This book was conceptualized with the vision of imparting up-to-date and integrated information in this field. To ensure the same, a matchless editorial board was set up. Every individual on the board went through rigorous rounds of assessment to prove their worth. After which they invested a large part of their time researching and compiling the most relevant data for our readers.

The editorial board has been involved in producing this book since its inception. They have spent rigorous hours researching and exploring the diverse topics which have resulted in the successful publishing of this book. They have passed on their knowledge of decades through this book. To expedite this challenging task, the publisher supported the team at every step. A small team of assistant editors was also appointed to further simplify the editing procedure and attain best results for the readers.

Apart from the editorial board, the designing team has also invested a significant amount of their time in understanding the subject and creating the most relevant covers. They scrutinized every image to scout for the most suitable representation of the subject and create an appropriate cover for the book.

The publishing team has been an ardent support to the editorial, designing and production team. Their endless efforts to recruit the best for this project, has resulted in the accomplishment of this book. They are a veteran in the field of academics and their pool of knowledge is as vast as their experience in printing. Their expertise and guidance has proved useful at every step. Their uncompromising quality standards have made this book an exceptional effort. Their encouragement from time to time has been an inspiration for everyone.

The publisher and the editorial board hope that this book will prove to be a valuable piece of knowledge for students, practitioners and scholars across the globe.

Index

Printed in the USA
CPSIA information can be obtained
at www.ICGtesting.com
JSHW051321221024
72173JS00006B/1281

9 798887 405452